ORTHOPEDIC CLINICS OF NORTH AMERICA

www.orthopedic.theclinics.com

Hot Topics in Orthopedic Surgery

April 2021 • Volume 52 • Number 2

ELSEVIER

1600 John F. Kennedy Boulevard • Suite 1800 • Philadelphia, Pennsylvania, 19103-2899.

http://www.orthopedic.theclinics.com

ORTHOPEDIC CLINICS OF NORTH AMERICA Volume 52, Number 2
April 2021 ISSN 0030-5898, ISBN-13: 978-0-323-83576-3

Editor: Lauren Boyle
Developmental Editor: Ann Gielou M. Posedio

Orthopedic Clinics of North America (ISSN 0030-5898) is published quarterly by Elsevier Inc., 360 Park Avenue South, New York, NY 10010-1710. Months of issue are January, April, July, and October. Business and Editorial Offices: 1600 John F. Kennedy Blvd., Suite 1800, Philadelphia, PA 19103-2899. Customer Service Office: 3251 Riverport Lane, Maryland Heights, MO 63043. Periodicals postage paid at New York, NY and additional mailing offices. Subscription prices are $347.00 per year for (US individuals), $1,003.00 per year for (US institutions), $411.00 per year (Canadian individuals), $1,028.00 per year (Canadian institutions), $476.00 per year (international individuals), $1,028.00 per year (international institutions), $100.00 per year (US students), $100.00 per year for (Canadian students), $220.00 per year for (international students). Foreign air speed delivery is included in all *Clinics* subscription prices. All prices are subject to change without notice. **POSTMASTER:** Send change of address to *Orthopedic Clinics of North America*, **Elsevier Health Sciences Division, Subscription Customer Service, 3251 Riverport Lane, Maryland Heights, MO 63043. Customer Service (orders, claims, online, change of address): Elsevier Health Sciences Division, Subscription Customer Service, 3251 Riverport Lane, Maryland Heights, MO 63043. Tel: 1-800-654-2452 (U.S. and Canada); 314-447-8871 (outside U.S. and Canada). Fax: 314-447-8029. E-mail:** journalscustomerservice-usa@elsevier.com **(for print support);** journalsonlinesupport-usa@elsevier.com **(for online support).**

Reprints. For copies of 100 or more, of articles in this publication, please contact the Commercial Reprints Department, Elsevier Inc., 360 Park Avenue South, New York, NY 10010-1710. Tel.: 212-633-3874; Fax: 212-633-3820; E-mail: reprints@elsevier.com.

Orthopedic Clinics of North America is covered in *MEDLINE/PubMed* (*Index Medicus*), *Cinahl, Excerpta Medica,* and *Cumulative Index to Nursing and Allied Health Literature.*

EDITORIAL BOARD

CONTRIBUTORS

AUTHORS

ADESHINA ADEYEMO, MD, BSN
Department of Bone and Joint, Penn State
Milton Hershey Medical Center, Hershey,
Pennsylvania, USA

CHARLOTTE ALLEN, MBChB, FRACS
Footbridge Clinic, Providence Healthcare,
University of British Columbia, Vancouver,
British Columbia, Canada

COURTNEY E. BAKER, MD
Resident, Department of Orthopedic Surgery,
Mayo Clinic, Rochester, Minnesota, USA

CASEY M. BELECKAS, MD, MSc
Department of Orthopedics, Indiana
University

MICHAEL J. BELTRAN, MD
Associate Professor, Department of
Orthopaedic Surgery, University of Cincinnati,
Cincinnati, Ohio, USA

NICHOLAS BERTHA, MD
Department of Bone and Joint, Penn State
Milton Hershey Medical Center, Hershey,
Pennsylvania, USA

ALEXANDER V. BOIWKA, MD
Department of Orthopedic Surgery,
McGovern Medical School, UTHealth,
Houston, Texas, USA

KIMBERLY M. BROTHERS, PhD
Arthritis and Arthroplasty Design Group,
Department of Orthopaedic Surgery, College
of Medicine, University of Pittsburgh,
Pittsburgh, Pennsylvania, USA

ZORAN BURSAC, PhD
Professor and Chair, Department of
Biostatistics, Florida International University,
Miami, Florida, USA

JAMES H. CALANDRUCCIO, MD
Department of Orthopaedic Surgery and
Biomedical Engineering, Campbell Clinic,

University of Tennessee Health Science
Center, Memphis, Tennessee, USA

JONATHAN CALLEGARI, DO
Southern Oregon Orthopedics, Medford,
Oregon, USA

J. CHRIS COETZEE, MD
Twin Cities Orthopedics, Eagan, Minnesota,
USA

PATRICK DENARD, MD
Southern Oregon Orthopedics, Medford,
Oregon, USA; Department of Orthopaedics
and Rehabilitation, Oregon Health & Science
University, Portland, Oregon, USA

KAREN J. DEREFINKO, PhD
Assistant Professor, Department of Preventive
Medicine and Department of Pharmacology,
Addiction Science, and Toxicology, University
of Tennessee Health Science Center,
Memphis, Tennessee, USA

TRAVIS A. DOERING, MD
Department of Orthopaedic Surgery and
Biomedical Engineering, Campbell Clinic,
University of Tennessee Health Science
Center, Memphis, Tennessee, USA

ADAM M. FREEDHAND, MD
Department of Orthopedic Surgery,
McGovern Medical School, UTHealth,
Houston, Texas, USA

MARK GLAZEBROOK, MD, MSc, PhD, Dip
Sports Med, FRCSC
Professor of Orthopaedics, Dalhouse
University, Queen Elizabeth II Hospital,
Halifax, Nova Scotia, Canada

ZHENGHUA GONG, MS
Data Analyst, Department of Biostatistics,
Florida International University, Miami,
Florida, USA

ALEXANDRA GRABRIELLI, MD
Arthritis and Arthroplasty Design Group,
Department of Orthopaedic Surgery, College
of Medicine, University of Pittsburgh,
Pittsburgh, Pennsylvania, USA

GEORGES HAIDAMOUS, MD
University of South Florida Morsani College of
Medicine, Florida Orthopedic Institute,
Foundation for Orthopedic Research and
Education, Tampa, Florida, USA

SHUYANG HAN, PhD
Department of Orthopedic Surgery,
McGovern Medical School, UTHealth,
Houston, Texas, USA

SARAH B. HAND, MPH, CCRP
Senior Research Project Coordinator,
Department of Preventive Medicine,
University of Tennessee Health Science
Center, Memphis, Tennessee, USA

POOYA HOSSEINZADEH, MD
Assistant Professor, Pediatric and Adolescent
Orthopaedic Surgery, Department of
Orthopaedic Surgery, Washington University
School of Medicine, St Louis, Missouri, USA

KAREN C. JOHNSON, MD, MPH
Chair and Endowed Professor, Department of
Preventive Medicine, University of Tennessee
Health Science Center, Memphis, Tennessee,
USA

ALEXANDRE LÄDERMANN, MD
Division of Orthopaedics and Trauma Surgery,
La Tour Hospital, Meyrin, Switzerland; Faculty
of Medicine, University of Geneva, Geneva 4,
Switzerland; Division of Orthopaedics and
Trauma Surgery, Department of Surgery,
Geneva University Hospitals, Geneva 14,
Switzerland

A. NOELLE LARSON, MD
Professor, Department of Orthopedic
Surgery, Mayo Clinic, Rochester, Minnesota,
USA

KENNETH B. MATHIS, MD
Department of Orthopedic Surgery,
McGovern Medical School, UTHealth,
Houston, Texas, USA

BENJAMIN M. MAUCK, MD
Department of Orthopaedic Surgery and
Biomedical Engineering, Campbell Clinic,

University of Tennessee Health Science
Center, Memphis, Tennessee, USA

REBECCA STONE McGAVER, MS, ATC
Twin Cities Orthopedics, Eagan, Minnesota,
USA

WILLIAM M. MIHALKO, MD, PhD
Professor and JR Hyde Chair of Excellence,
Department of Orthopaedic Surgery and
Biomedical Engineering, Chair, Joint
Graduate Program in Biomedical Engineering,
Campbell Clinic, University of Tennessee
Health Science Center, Memphis, Tennessee,
USA

TODD A. MILBRANDT, MD, MS
Professor, Department of Orthopedic
Surgery, Mayo Clinic, Rochester, Minnesota,
USA

PHILIP C. NOBLE, PhD
Department of Orthopedic Surgery,
McGovern Medical School, UTHealth,
Houston, Texas, USA

KEVIN J. PERRY, MD, DPT
Department of Bone and Joint, Penn State
Milton Hershey Medical Center, Hershey,
Pennsylvania, USA

CAMERON PHILLIPS, MD
Southern Oregon Orthopedics, Medford,
Oregon, USA

FERNANDO RADUAN, MD
Twin Cities Orthopedics, Eagan, Minnesota,
USA

DAVID RODRIGUEZ-QUINTANA, MD
Department of Orthopedic Surgery,
McGovern Medical School, UTHealth,
Houston, Texas, USA

MAKSIM A. SHLYKOV, MD, MS
Orthopaedic Surgery Resident, Department of
Orthopaedic Surgery, Washington University
School of Medicine/Barnes-Jewish Hospital, St
Louis, Missouri, USA

JAN P. SZATKOWSKI, MD, MBA
Department of Orthopedics, Indiana
University, IU Health

SHANE TRACY, PA-C
Southern Oregon Orthopedics, Medford,
Oregon, USA

GARY UPDEGROVE, MD
Department of Bone and Joint, Penn State
Milton Hershey Medical Center, Hershey,
Pennsylvania, USA

KENNETH L. URISH, MD, PhD
Arthritis and Arthroplasty Design Group,
Department of Orthopaedic Surgery, College
of Medicine, University of Pittsburgh,
Pittsburgh, Pennsylvania, USA

ANDREA VELJKOVIC, MD, MPH, BComm,
FAOA, FRCSC
Associate Clinical Professor, Department of
Orthopaedics, Footbridge Clinic, St Pauls
Hospital, Providence Healthcare, University of
British Columbia, Vancouver, British
Columbia, Canada

PETER R. WASKY, MD
Orthopaedic Surgery Resident, Department of
Orthopaedic Surgery, University of Cincinnati,
Cincinnati, Ohio, USA

ALASTAIR YOUNGER, MBChB, MSc, ChM,
FRCSC
Footbridge Clinic, Professor of Orthopaedics,
St Pauls Hospital, Providence Healthcare,
University of British Columbia, Vancouver,
British Columbia, Canada

JASON ZLOTNICKI, MD
Arthritis and Arthroplasty Design Group,
Department of Orthopaedic Surgery, College
of Medicine, University of Pittsburgh,
Pittsburgh, Pennsylvania, USA

CONTENTS

Knee and Hip Reconstruction

The success of total knee arthroplasty (TKA) depends on restoration of the stability and biomechanical efficiency of the native knee. The emergence of robotic surgical technologies has greatly increased the precision and reproducibility. We discuss contemporary robotic TKA systems by reviewing the features of the individual platforms, their accuracy, and the clinical outcomes. While early results suggest significant gains in patient outcomes, long-term evidence is still awaited from multicenter prospective clinical trials. Moreover, advances in this technology are needed to address knee laxity while individualizing the functional performance of each patient's new joint.

In orthopedic infections, hydrogen peroxide, povidone-iodine, and chlorhexidine are added to irrigants to prevent and treat infection. A larger body of evidence supports their use as a prophylaxis to prevent infection as compared with treating infection. Biofilm has a high tolerance to antimicrobials induced by oxidative stress. This review examines some of the most widely reported interventions. Techniques for irrigation and extended oral antibiotic regimens are presented. The role of irrigants in periprosthetic joint infection for treatment of planktonic and biofilm bacteria is discussed. The newest advances in the field of adjuvants for prevention of periprosthetic joint infection are presented.

Orthopedic surgeries are associated with the prescription of more narcotics than any other surgical specialty, particularly for total knee replacement (TKR) surgery. The authors examined controlled substance prescriptions following TKR surgery in a sample of 560 TKR patients. Results indicated that of all the 5164 prescriptions documented on the controlled substance monitoring database, 64% were for opioid medications. More than half of the patients received controlled substances from both the surgery site provider and a nonsurgery site provider in the year following surgery. The authors recommend that providers consider the possibility of outside prescribing when prescribing opioid analgesic.

> Several articles in the literature discuss the positive results of converting a painful ankle fusion to an ankle replacement. Our results confirm that in well-selected cases a conversion to a total ankle replacement is not only possible, but also significantly improves quality of life and reduces pain. The outcome of a total ankle replacement after an ankle fusion depends to a degree on the method of fusion. Less destructive fusion that is arthroscopic has better results than conventional transfibular open fusions. Absence of a fibula should be an absolute contraindication for a conversion.

HOT TOPICS IN ORTHOPEDIC SURGERY

FORTHCOMING ISSUES

July 2021
Common Complications in Orthopedic
Surgery
Michael J. Beebe, Clayton C. Bettin, Tyler J.
Brolin, James H. Calandruccio, Benjamin J. Grear,
Benjamin M. Mauck, William M. Mihalko, Benjamin
Sheffer, David D. Spence, Patrick C. Toy, and John
C. Weinlein, *Editors*

October 2021
Fracture Care
Michael J. Beebe, Clayton C. Bettin, Tyler J.
Brolin, James H. Calandruccio, Christopher T.
Cosgrove, Benjamin J. Grear, Benjamin M. Mauck,
William M. Mihalko, Benjamin Sheffer, David D.
Spence, Kirk M. Thompson, and Patrick C. Toy,
Editors

RECENT ISSUES

January 2021
Education and Professional Development in
Orthopedics
Michael J. Beebe, Clayton C. Bettin, Tyler J.
Brolin, James H. Calandruccio, Benjamin J. Grear,
Benjamin M. Mauck, William M. Mihalko, Jeffrey R.
Sawyer, David D. Spence, Patrick C. Toy, and John
C. Weinlein, *Editors*

October 2020
Sports-Related Injuries
Michael J. Beebe, Clayton C. Bettin, Tyler J.
Brolin, James H. Calandruccio, Benjamin J. Grear,
Benjamin M. Mauck, William M. Mihalko, Jeffrey R.
Sawyer, David D. Spence, Patrick C. Toy, and John
C. Weinlein, *Editors*

SERIES OF RELATED INTEREST

Foot and Ankle Clinics
https://www.foot.theclinics.com/
Clinics in Sports Medicine
https://www.sportsmed.theclinics.com/
Hand Clinics
https://www.hand.theclinics.com/
Physical Medicine and Rehabilitation Clinics
https://www.pmr.theclinics.com/

PREFACE

Hot Topics in Orthopedics

Orthopedic surgeons have always been great innovators and inventors, witness the plethora of techniques and devices for fracture fixation, joint replacement, and deformity correction. Never satisfied with the status quo and convinced that better outcomes can be obtained, orthopedic surgeons continue to develop techniques for improving patient function and decreasing adverse events. This issue of *Orthopedic Clinics of North America* contains many excellent introductions to some of the recent developments in orthopedic surgery.

Dr Han and colleagues explain the advantages of robotic systems for total knee replacement and discuss contemporary robotic total knee arthroplasty (TKA) systems that have gained or are pending Food and Drug Administration approval. They review the features of the individual robotic platforms, their accuracy in achieving the surgeon's preoperative plan, and the resulting clinical outcome in terms of patient function and satisfaction. Periprosthetic infection is a dreaded complication of total joint replacement surgery, and investigations continue to identify methods to decrease its frequency. Drs Zlontnicki and colleagues discuss the addition of hydrogen peroxide, povidone-iodine, and chlorhexidine to irrigants to prevent and treat infection and note that a large body of evidence supports their use as prophylaxis to prevent infection as compared with treating infection. After finding that over half of TKA patients received controlled substances from both the surgery site provider and a nonsurgery site provider in the year following surgery, Dr Derefinko and colleagues caution that orthopedic surgeons should consider the possibility of outside prescribing when prescribing opioid analgesic.

Treatment of fractures has been the focus of many and varied devices and techniques. Drs Wasky and Beltran describe the use of "extreme" intramedullary nailing and less-invasive plating of lower-extremity periarticular fractures, noting that the indications for the use of extreme nailing is multifactorial and is based on fracture pattern, condition of the soft tissues, the medical condition of the patient, and the importance of earlier or immediate weight-bearing. Nontraditional methods of fibular fixation, such as minimally invasive methods, are described and discussed by Drs Beleckas and Szatkowski. They note the effectiveness of these techniques for ensuring a superior prognosis for ankle fractures.

Drs Hosseinzadeh and Shlykov discuss the growing practice of dual fellowships for pediatric sports medicine specialists and its impact on patient care and training patterns. Drs Baker, Milbrandt, and Larson review the translational science foundation, early to mid-term clinical reports, and future directions for the nonfusion technique of anterior vertebral body tethering for adolescent idiopathic scoliosis.

Advances in diagnosis and management for common complaints and complex injuries of the hand and wrist, including volar locked plating of distal radial fractures, WALANT (wide awake local anesthesia no tourniquet) for outpatient procedures, and techniques for tendon and nerve repair and reconstruction, are described and discussed by Dr Doering. The review article by Dr Callegari and colleagues summarizes the effects of modern reverse shoulder prostheses on outcomes. In a detailed review of the literature, Dr Adeyemo and colleagues found that no definitive answers are available regarding best practice for proximal humeral fractures, but there is literature to guide operative decision making and implant selection based on both patient- and surgeon-specific factors.

Dr Allen and colleagues noted that, with growing demand for foot and ankle services, the roles of podiatrists and orthopedic surgeons are increasingly overlapping and need to be defined. They examined the overlapping scope of practice

Orthop Clin N Am 52 (2021) xv–xvi
https://doi.org/10.1016/j.ocl.2021.02.001
0030-5898/21/© 2021 Published by Elsevier Inc.

of each of the groups and compared the relative costs and outcomes associated with each. The conversion of an ankle arthrodesis to a total ankle arthroplasty was long thought to be extremely difficult if not impossible, but Drs Coetzee, Raduan, and McGaver determined that in well-selected cases conversion to a total ankle replacement not only is possible but also significantly improves quality of life and reduces pain.

The contributors and I hope this information will assist you in making the treatment choices for your patients that will obtain optimal outcomes.

Frederick M. Azar, MD
Department of Orthopaedic Surgery &
Biomedical Engineering
University of Tennessee–Campbell Clinic
1211 Union Avenue, Suite 510
Memphis, TN 38104, USA

E-mail address:
fazar@campbellclinic.com

Knee and Hip Reconstruction

Contemporary Robotic Systems in Total Knee Arthroplasty

A Review of Accuracy and Outcomes

Shuyang Han, PhD[1], David Rodriguez-Quintana, MD[2],
Adam M. Freedhand, MD[2], Kenneth B. Mathis, MD[2],
Alexander V. Boiwka, MD[2], Philip C. Noble, PhD*,[1]

KEYWORDS

- Total knee arthroplasty • Robotic surgery • Computer-assisted surgery
- Component positioning

KEY POINTS

- The success of total knee arthroplasty (TKA), both in the short-term and long-term, depends on restoration of both the stability and biomechanical efficiency of the native knee. This necessitates correct positioning and alignment of the prosthetic components, matched to the anatomy and soft tissue properties of each individual patient at the time of surgery.
- There is general consensus that the outcome of TKA achieved using conventional manual instrumentation are highly variable and dependent on the skill and experience of the operating surgeon. This has led to the increasing adoption of computer-based technologies, most prominently surgical navigation and robotic surgical systems.
- The robotic assistance in positioning cutting tools and performing bone cuts enables surgeons to achieve idealized execution of preoperative planning, which has greatly increased the precision and reproducibility in the placement of prostheses.
- Although early results suggest significant gains in patient outcomes using robotic technologies, long-term evidence is still awaited from multicenter prospective clinical trials. Moreover, as most of these systems are directed to positioning and alignment of both the joint and the tibial and femoral components, and not the functional stability of the prosthetic knee, advances in this technology are needed to address knee laxity while individualizing the functional performance of each patient's new joint.

INTRODUCTION

The critical determinants of successful, durable total knee arthroplasty (TKA) are correct positioning of the implanted components, acceptable alignment of the knee, and restoration of joint stability during functional activities. However, the success in achieving target values of these parameters varies extensively between surgeons, which has led to interest in computer-assisted technologies to standardize the technical aspects of the procedure. In the early days of computer-assisted surgery, the role of technology was limited to surgical navigation. This information was used to guide the surgeon in manual placement of cutting guides as well as providing information concerning gap opening and limb alignment following placement of the implanted components. Since this time, robotic

Department of Orthopedic Surgery, McGovern Medical School, UTHealth-Houston, 5420 West Loop South, Suite 1300, Houston, TX 77401, USA
[1]Present address: 5420 West Loop South, Suite 1300, Bellaire, TX 77401.
[2]Present address: 5420 West Loop South, Suite 2400, Bellaire, TX 77401.
* Corresponding author.
E-mail address: philipnoble66@gmail.com

Orthop Clin N Am 52 (2021) 83–92
https://doi.org/10.1016/j.ocl.2020.12.001

systems have become available to implement the surgeon's surgical plan and provide confirmation of component placement and knee function intraoperatively. In this study, we review robotic TKA systems that are commercially available, and examine the published evidence documenting the effectiveness of these technologies in improving the accuracy and reliability in component position, joint alignment, and patient-reported outcomes.

Robotic surgical systems can be divided into 3 categories based on the degree of control provided to the operating surgeon: active/autonomous, semi-active, and passive.[1,2] In active systems, the robot autonomously executes the preplanned surgical procedure without physical guidance from the surgeon. Semi-active systems provide intraoperative auditory (beeping), tactile (vibration), or visual feedback to the surgeon to assist the surgeon in performing the bone cuts and positioning the components more accurately. In passive systems, the role of the robotic system is to provide guidance and position instruments (eg, cutting blocks) while all or part of the procedure itself is carried out under the surgeon's direct control.

Robotic systems are also differentiated by the source of data used to create the individualized surgical plan. These are classified as either "image-based" or "imageless." In image-based systems, a 3-dimensional (3D) computer model of the patient's bony anatomy is created from preoperative imaging data, including plain radiographs and data derived from computed tomography

(CT) or MRI. The 3D model of the patient's bony anatomy is then used to determine the depth and location of the bony resections, the size of the implanted components, and their alignment with respect to the femur and tibia according to the patient's unique skeletal morphology (Fig. 1).[3]

To replicate these resections during surgery, the models and the patient's joint surfaces must be spatially matched (ie, "registered ") before the robot can execute the preoperative surgical plan. In imageless systems, these steps are performed intraoperatively by predicting the surface coordinates of the femur and tibia using accessible areas of the bony surfaces and various anatomic landmarks. This information is used as a basis for predicting the patient's bony morphology by scaling preexisting anatomic models.

CONTEMPORARY ROBOTIC SYSTEMS FOR TOTAL KNEE ARTHROPLASTY AND SURGICAL OUTCOMES

Many robotic TKA platforms have been developed and used in clinical settings worldwide, resulting in a dramatic increase in peer-reviewed publications.[1,4–7] Within the United States, the Food and Drug Administration (FDA) has given approval for the use of a variety of robotic TKA systems with varying features and functions (Table 1). We now review the features of the individual robotic platforms, their accuracy in achieving the surgeon's preoperative plan, and the resulting clinical outcome in terms of patient function and satisfaction.

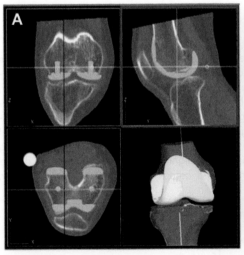
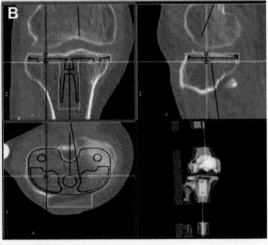

Fig. 1. Image-based preoperative planning to determine the size and alignment of the femoral (A) and tibial (B) components. (From Song EK, Seon JK, Park SJ, et al. Simultaneous bilateral total knee arthroplasty with robotic and conventional techniques: a prospective, randomized study. Knee Surg Sports Traumatol Arthrosc 2011;19(7):1069-1076; with permission.)

Table 1
Historic and contemporary robotic systems used for TKA

Robotic System	Resection Type	Preop Imaging	Control	FDA Approval Date
Mako	Semi-active	Preop CT	Haptic feedback	Aug. 2015
Omnibotics	Passive	Imageless	Manual (robotically positioned cutting guide)	Sept. 2017
Navio	Semi-active	Imageless	Robotic-assisted non-haptic	Jun. 2017
Rosa	Semi-active	Preop radiograph or imageless	Manual (robotically positioned cutting guide)	Jan. 2019
Robodoc/ TSolution One	Active	Preop CT	Autonomous control	Oct. 2019
CORI	Semi-active	Imageless	Robotic-assisted non-haptic	Jul. 2020
Orthotaxy	Semi-active	Imageless	-	
MBARS	Active	Imageless	Autonomous control	
CASPAR	Active	Preop CT	Autonomous control	
Acrobot/Sculptor	Semi-active	Preop CT	Active-constraint	
PiGalileo	Passive	Imageless	Manual	

Abbreviations: CT, computed tomography; Preop, preoperative; TKA, total knee arthroplasty.

The Mako Robotic Arm System

The Mako (Stryker, Mahwah, NJ) robotic arm system is an image-based semi-active system widely used in robotic-assisted Unicompartmental knee arthroplasty (UKA) and Total hip arthroplasty (THA). The Mako TKA system was approved by the FDA in 2015. As an image-based system, a preoperative, patient-specific CT model of each patient's knee is created to enable selection of the appropriate component sizes and locations. Intraoperatively, the bony models, as well as the planned implant components, are registered to the patient's anatomy by digitizing bony landmarks. The patient's knee is brought through a range of motion to assess deformity and laxity.

The collateral ligaments are then tensioned in extension and flexion and the gap values captured for evaluation. These gap values are then corrected to achieve correct alignment and ligament balance through manipulating the preplanned component positions before bone resection. Once the desired 3D plan has been created, the corresponding cuts can be made with a conventional surgical saw mounted on the robotic arm. Haptic feedback helps the surgeon to control the force and direction of saw blade within the confines of the predefined resection zone, thereby protecting soft tissue structures such as the medial collateral ligament and posterior cruciate ligament.[1,4–6]

Many studies have investigated the Mako robotic system in terms of its accuracy and cost-effectiveness, clinical outcomes, and patient satisfaction. At 6-month follow-up, Marchand and colleagues[8] compared the outcomes of 20 Mako-assisted and 20 manual TKAs in terms of pain score, functional score, and patient satisfaction. The robotic cohort showed significantly lower pain score (3 ± 3 vs 5 ± 3, $P<.05$) and higher patient satisfaction (14 ± 8 vs 7 ± 8 points, $P<.05$). In a prospective study of 150 Mako-assisted and 102 manual TKAs,[9] the robotic cohort had equal or greater improvements in 9 of 10 components of the Knee Society Score at 3 months postoperatively, including the functional activities score, the total symptom score, and the satisfaction and expectation scores.

In terms of coronal alignment, the Mako system has demonstrated accuracy in correcting knees with deformities of 9° to 15° varus or valgus.[10] Sultan and colleagues[11] compared the posterior condylar offset ratio (PCOR) and the Insall-Salvati Index (ISI) in 43 Mako TKAs and 39 manual TKAs at 4 to 6 weeks postoperatively. The robotic cohort had smaller mean differences in PCOR (0.49 vs 0.53, $P = .024$) than the manual group, which has been shown to correlate with better ROM at 1 year after TKA. The number of patients with ISI outside of the normal range was also lower in the robotic cohort (4 vs 12), that is, patients in the robotic group are less likely to develop restricted flexion and overall ROM. In addition, there are data showing smaller errors in bone cuts and component positioning relative to preoperative plans following use of the Mako system.[12]

As with most new surgical technologies, there is a learning curve associated with the Mako TKA system. An analysis of 240 Mako-assisted TKAs performed by 2 surgeons indicated that the operative procedure was significantly longer during the first 20 cases. Thereafter, operative times were comparable between robotic TKA and conventional manual TKA.[13] In another study, Kayani and colleagues[14] assessed the learning curve using a set of surrogate operative and radiographic markers in 60 consecutive conventional TKAs and 60 Mako-assisted TKAs. The results suggested a learning curve of 7 cases for operative time and surgical team anxiety level. Moreover, there was no penalty in changing from conventional to robotic instrumentation in terms of femoral and tibial implant positioning, limb alignment, PCOR, posterior tibial slope, or restoration of the joint line.[14]

Adoption of the robotic system is associated with substantial installation and maintenance costs, as well as costs related to the cost of disposable accessories, preoperative imaging, and training of the surgical team. In 2015, the estimated upfront costs of the Mako UKA platform as well as service contract costs were $1.362 million.[15] However, Cool and colleagues[16] calculated a 90-day episode-of-care cost of 519 Mako-assisted TKA and 2595 conventional TKA, including the index costs, index lengths-of-stay, discharge dispositions, and readmissions. The study showed that the episode-of-care costs were US$2391 less for robotic TKA ($18568 vs $20960, $P<.0001$) in 2018 dollars.[16] Over 90% of patients in both cohorts utilized post-acute services, with robotic TKA accruing fewer costs than manual TKA ($5234 vs $6978; $P<.0001$).

OMNIBotics

The OMNIBotics (OMNIlife Science Inc., East Taunton, MA) implantation system is an imageless platform that consists of a bone modeling module (Bone Morphing), a ligament balancing robot (BalanceBot), and a resection robot (OMNIBot). A patient-specific 3D model of the joint is created intraoperatively using bone morphing technology, which registers sparse point data with a statistical deformable model.[17] The BalanceBot is used to measure ligament tension and the resultant gaps throughout the midflexion range. Then, taking into account the mechanical axis, the 3D bone morphology, and

the tibiofemoral gaps, the implant position is planned on the navigation system, and the BalanceBot is mounted to the femur fixation base and locked into varus/valgus alignment and internal/external rotation. A single cutting guide is then aligned in the sagittal plane for each of the 5 femoral cuts to allow the surgeon to perform the bony resections.[18,19]

Several studies have shown increased efficiency and accuracy of bone resection in cases performed with the robotic cutting guide, which was named iBlock at the time.[20–23] Suero and colleagues[20] compared 30 TKAs using iBlock with 64 manual TKAs. Within the robotic cases, they found reduced variability in limb alignment (standard deviation: 1.7° vs 2.7°, $P = .0091$) and tourniquet time (76 min vs 91 min, $P = .008$). In another study, the same investigators evaluated the accuracy and postoperative limb alignment in 100 TKAs using iBlock for femoral resection.[22] The femoral and tibial component alignment was within 3° of neutral alignment in 98% of cases and final limb alignment was restored to within 3° in 87% of cases.[22] In a cadaveric study, it was found that the iBlock was associated with a substantial reduction from 13.8 min to 5.5 min in the time required for femoral preparation ($P<.001$) while achieving more accurate bone resections in all anatomic planes.[21] Similar findings regarding bone resection were also reported by Ponder and colleagues.[23]

Regarding soft tissue balancing, Koenig and colleagues[24] compared the final intraoperative coronal balance throughout 0° to 90° of flexion in 27 OmniBotics-assisted TKAs and 25 manual TKAs. There was a statistically significant difference in the gaps between the 2 groups at 60 to 90° of flexion. Overall, 78% to 86% of robotic cases were balanced to within 2 mm compared with 65% to 76% without robotic assistance.

Revenga and colleagues[25,26] and Hernandez-Vaquero and colleagues[27] compared the European Knee Society Score (KSS), Western Ontario and McMaster Universities Osteoarthritis Index (WOMAC), and Short Form (SF)-12 scores of 892 patients (343 OmniBotics vs 549 Conventional) at 2 years of follow-up. The OminiBotics group showed greater improvement in the KSS score; the WOMAC pain, stiffness, and function subscores; and the SF-12 physical function score. Similarly, Keggi and colleagues[28,29] reported early patient satisfaction of OmniBotics-assisted TKAs in 29 knees. All patients were either "Fully Satisfied" (86%) or "Partly Satisfied" (14%) with their surgery. In an ongoing prospective study comparing OmniBotics-assisted TKA and conventional TKA,[19] the KSS satisfaction score at 6 months postoperative improved by 19 points in the robotic group, twice the improvement of those receiving conventional TKA. At 1-year follow-up, there was greater improvement in knee function, pain reduction, satisfaction, and quality of life.

There is a learning curve associated with the use of iBlock. Compared with conventional TKA, the robotic TKA took an average of 15 extra minutes during the first 10 cases and 5 extra minutes during the second 10 without compromising accuracy.[22] It was also found that, after the first 7 cases, the operative time (skin-to-skin) decreased by 27 minutes from 84 to 57 minutes.[28,29] In contrast, other studies have shown that robotic assistance extended the duration of TKA by an average of only 3.3 minutes.[25–27] In addition, Licini and Meneghini[30] reported a reduced rate of blood loss ($P = .02$), drop in hemoglobin levels ($P = .001$), and estimated total blood loss ($P = .001$) in cases performed with the assistance of this robotic system, compared with conventional instrumentation.

The Navio Surgical System

Navio (Smith & Nephew, London, UK) is a handheld, imageless, semi-active robotic system that combines surgical planning, navigation, and intraoperative visualization. The system has been approved by the FDA for TKA as well as unicondylar and patellofemoral knee arthroplasty.[5–7] The Navio system is composed of a robotically controlled handheld burr and a point probe, which is integrated with a passive infrared camera tracking system and a surgeon-controlled graphical user interface.[31] These components are mounted on a mobile computer cart. Navio relies on intraoperative 3D images to create a virtual model of the osseous knee and to guide bone resection. Unlike the Mako system, the Navio system does not rely on haptic feedback. Rather, it has a handheld end-cutting burr that can extend and retract during the procedure so that only the planned bone is removed.

Specifically, the system monitors the position of the burring tool with respect to the patient's lower extremity, and when the edge of the desired bone resection volume is approached, the burr tip retracts to avoid over-resection.[1] The Navio TKA system is compatible with a variety of Smith & Nephew knee replacements, including the Journey-II, Legion, and Genesis implant designs.

The Navio system has demonstrated high accuracy for bone preparation and gap balancing in TKA. In the first attempt to evaluate its accuracy in TKA, Casper and colleagues[31] used the robotic system in 18 cadaveric knees, and reported an overall error in the varus/valgus orientation of the femur of $-0.1° \pm 0.9°$, a tibial varus/valgus error of $-0.2° \pm 0.9°$, and an error of $-0.2° \pm 1.3°$ in the posterior slope of the tibial component. However, the femoral implant flexion/extension error reached $-2.0° \pm 2.2°$. Jaramaz and colleagues[32] measured the translational, angular, and rotational differences between the planned and achieved positions of components implanted in cadaveric and synthetic bones with the Navio TKA system. The root mean square (RMS) errors of femoral varus/valgus, rotation and distal resection were 0.7°, 0.7°, and 0.86 mm, respectively. The RMS errors of tibial posterior slope, varus/valgus, and resection depth were 0.88°, 0.69°, and 0.68 mm, respectively, which suggests that the Navio system provides relatively accurate implementation of the surgical plan. At the time of writing, there are limited data available in terms of the incidence of complications, patient outcomes, or the length of the learning curve associated with the use of the Navio robotic system.

The CORI Surgical System

The CORI surgical system (Smith & Nephew) is an imageless portable robotic system for use in total and unicompartmental knee arthroplasty. The CORI system offers image-free mapping of bone geometry, intraoperative planning and gap assessment, and confirmation of alignment and knee balance after the surgery.

As the most recent addition to the range of commercially available robotic knee instrumentation systems, the CORI system has been developed to operate within a smaller footprint than earlier generations of robotic systems. This has been combined with a focus on increased efficiency of workflow through improvements in the speed of the surgical navigation through the use of higher-speed camera technology. The rate of bone removal has also been increased through the use of higher-speed cutting burrs. The CORI robotic system has been configured to support a broad range of knee prostheses, all manufactured by Smith & Nephew, including the Journey-II, Anthem, Legion, and Genesis-II total knee designs.

Gregori and colleagues[33] used the system in 92 cases of medial unicompartmental knee arthroplasty and reported that the coronal mechanical axis alignment of the knee was restored to within 3° of the planned value in 89% patients. The RMS errors in implant position were: femoral coronal alignment (2.6°), tibial coronal alignment (2.9°), and tibial slope (2.9°). Since the CORI system was approved by the FDA in 2020, data regarding the outcome, satisfaction, and cost-effectiveness of this technology in performing TKA has yet to be reported.

Rosa Knee System

The Rosa Knee system (Zimmer Biomet, Warsaw, IN) gained FDA approval in January 2019. This robotic system offers a computer software program to convert 2D X-ray images into a 3D patient-specific bone model, allowing virtual planning on implant positioning and ligament balancing before execution.

The principle of the system is simple: a manual cutting jig is positioned in the desired location by the Rosa robotic arm, as determined by the operative plan, allowing the surgeon to perform the bone cuts using manual instruments.[5,34,35] The Rosa knee system supports the Persona, Vanguard, and NexGen implant families.

With respect to the accuracy of the Rosa system, Parratte and colleagues[34] investigated the depth and angle of bony resection in a recent study of 30 cadaveric knees. It was found that, on average, the frontal, and sagittal alignment of bone cuts performed using the Rosa system were within 1° ± 1° of planned values. Except for the femoral sagittal angle (−0.95° ± 0.88°), there was no difference between the planned angles and the measured values. In terms of the resection thickness, there was no difference between the planned and measured values at all but 2 locations, the distal femoral condyle (0.3 mm) and medial tibial plateau (0.66 mm). In addition, Seidenstein and colleagues[35] compared the accuracy and reproducibility of the Rosa Knee system in 14 robotic TKAs (7 cadaveric specimens) and 20 conventional TKAs (10 cadaveric specimens). The robotic group demonstrated greater accuracy in achieving target values, with fewer outliers than conventional instrumentation, with 100% versus 75% of cases within 3° and 93% versus 60% within 2° of the targeted hip-knee-ankle angle.

Robodoc and THINK-TSolution One Surgical System

The Robodoc system was first designed by Curexo Technology (Fremont, CA) for preparation of the femoral canal for cementless THA. The Robodoc system was then modified for use in TKA procedures and installed in Germany after being approved for sale in the European Union.[36] In 2014, Curexo Technology changed its name to THINK Surgical Inc and introduced a newer version of the Robodoc system for use in TKA, named the TSolution One surgical system after approval by the US FDA on October 8, 2019.

The TSolution One Surgical System is an autonomous milling system based on preoperative CT scans. It consists of 3 components: a 3D preoperative planning workstation, a surgical robot, and a computer control unit. For preoperative planning, computer models derived through CT scans of patients are used in a virtual surgery to determine the desired mechanical axis and implant sizes with the help of anatomic landmarks. The system has an open library of legally marketed implants for the US and international markets. The surgical plan is then loaded to the TSolution One Surgical System before surgery. Intraoperatively, recovery markers and bone movement monitors are rigidly attached to the femur and tibia to allow surface registration of the models. Then, the robotic system executes the preoperative cut plan, without active feedback from the operating surgeon.

The results of the first 100 cases performed with the original Robodoc TKA system were reported by Börner and colleagues in 2004 and showed that the accuracy of bone resection was sufficient for surgical applications with no cases of varus malpositioning of the knee postoperatively.[37] The accuracy of the system in replicating the preoperative plan was also demonstrated in a 25-patient study in which the mean deviation in coronal mechanical alignment was −0.4 ± 1.7°, with 100% accuracy in prediction of component sizes implanted intraoperatively.[38] In a 4-year follow-up of 72 knees, Park and Lee[39] reported differences in the coronal femoral angle (97.7° vs 95.6°, $P<.01$), sagittal femoral angle (0.2° vs 4.2°, $P<.01$), and sagittal tibial angles (85.5° vs 89.7°, $P<.01$) of robotic versus conventional TKA. At 10-year follow-up, Yang and colleagues[40] reported that the robotic cohort had significantly fewer outliers in terms of excessive deviation from the mechanical axis (8.5% vs 31%) and fewer radiolucent lines (0% vs 14%) than the conventional TKA group. Contrarily, at a mean of 13 years' follow-up, the femorotibial angle, femoral component position, tibial component position, joint line, and posterior femoral condylar offset were not different between robotic-assisted TKAs and conventional TKAs ($P>.05$).[41]

In terms of improvements in clinical outcomes after TKR performed using the Robodoc system, Yang and colleagues[40] reported no significant differences in Hospital for Special Surgery (HSS) score (88.7 vs 87.2, $P = .79$), WOMAC score (7.6 vs 11.5, $P = .12$), Visual Analog Scale pain score (1.1 vs 1.2, $P = .51$), and ROM (132.6° vs 131.0°, $P = .92$) at 10-year follow-up. Similar conclusions were reached by Cho and colleagues[42] who recently reported outcomes in 155 Robodoc TKAs versus 196 conventional NexGen TKAs, at a minimum 10 years OF follow-up. They reported no difference in WOMAC, Oxford Knee Score, KSS, or SF-12 scores. In addition, at a mean of 13 years' follow-up, Kim and colleagues[41] found that there were no differences in KSS, WOMAC, ROM, UCLA patient activity scores between robotic and conventional TKA groups. In contrast, Liow and colleagues[43] reported higher SF-36 quality-of-life measures in 31 robotic TKAs than in 29 conventional jig-based TKAs at 2-year follow-up.

In terms of the survivorship of robotic-assisted and conventional TKAs was not significantly different at 5 years (98.5% vs 97.6%, $P>.05$),[40] 10 years (97.1% and 92.3%, $P>.05$),[40] and 15 years (98% vs 98%, $P = .972$).[41] In addition, there was an obvious learning curve associated with the Robodoc TKA system, with operating time decreasing from 130 minutes for the first case to an average of 90 to 100 minutes after 27 cases.[3,37,38] Overall, robotic-assisted implantation increased operative times by approximately 25 minutes (95 vs 70 minutes).[3] Jacofsky and Allen[1] noted that the time needed for planning, registration, and milling is greater than many other robotic systems.

Orthotaxy Robotic Total Knee Arthroplasty System

The Orthotaxy TKA system is developed by Johnson & Johnson/DePuy-Synthes and currently pending FDA approval. Unlike other surgical robotic systems, it is reported that the Orthotaxy system is compact (ie, the size of a shoebox) and is attached to the operating table.[44] The system does not require preoperative CT imaging. Like other semi-active systems, the cutting guide is locked into position according to preoperative planning, allowing the surgeon to perform all bony cuts using an oscillating saw. Because the Orthotaxy robot will not require surgeons to use disposable instruments, savings compared with other robotic systems are projected to range from $1500 to $2500 per procedure. Moreover, the system is designed to be used without the assistance of an additional technician, potentially saving additional cost. This might be associated with a short learning curve.[44]

DISCUSSION

In this study we evaluated contemporary robotic systems for TKA in the United States and made mention, with the information available, of the robotic systems that are pending FDA approval.

These systems vary in function and features. There are robotic devices that are active, semi-active, and passive. Some are imageless and others are image-based technologies. All of the systems with the exception of TSolution One are closed platforms that are programmed for use with the implants of single manufacturers. It appears that there are benefits and disadvantages to some of the features discussed, as highlighted by many of the cited studies.[1,4,6]

The benefit of improved radiographic alignment and accuracy of component placement in concurrence with the surgical plan is improved compared with manually instrumented TKA in all the robotic platforms evaluated, although there was some variation. Although this was not necessarily believed to be clinically relevant until recently, it has become apparent through the analysis of registry data of computer-navigated TKA, that component position has an important influence on survivorship. When you look at the studies on robotic systems that provide a joint/ligament balancing feature (eg, Mako and Omni-Botics), you begin to see improvements in functional outcome scores and other clinically important findings such as decreased blood loss and potentially reduced cost,[11,25,26,30] in addition to improved clinical alignment.[20,22]

It must be recognized that most robotic systems implement preoperative plans based on the positions and relative alignment of the femur, tibia, and patella within each patient's diseased knee. However, once the surgical site is exposed, the menisci and osteophytes have been resected, along with one or both cruciate ligaments, these relationships will not generally correspond to the ideal position and alignment of the prosthetic components required to restore ideal stability and function. Moreover, unless all 3 bones of the knee are resurfaced using custom components, the surgeon must attempt to optimize knee function using implants that are an average approximation of each patient's native morphology, even if perfectly aligned and positioned. Few systems assess the laxity of the final prosthetic joint in a standardized fashion by measuring the kinematic response of the joint during application of set forces and moments. Some robotic systems indicate changes in medial and lateral joint opening or the separation of landmarks at preset flexion angles or during a continuous arc of motion under the surgeon's manual control. Others allow the surgeon to assess the varus/valgus laxity of the intact and replaced knee manually; however, during these procedures joint loading is not standardized. Clearly, significant advancement of surgical navigation and robotic technology is awaited to enable ideal values of the laxity of the prosthetic knee to be defined, planned, created, and confirmed using the tools that are presently available.

These findings raise the important question, "when is it appropriate to use robotics in TKA?" It would seem that it would almost always be appropriate to use a device that can provide for better, more consistent radiographic alignment coupled with a knee that has balanced ligaments to benefit the patient. The more difficult question becomes when not to use it? Perhaps in cases in which the bone quality is so poor that pin site fracture risk is a concern, or where the patient has a unique deformity such that enough data cannot be generated to perform the surgery robotically. These cases typically have severe contracture or massive articular aberrations in which bone registration may not be possible.

Robotic assistance in TKA is still in its introductory phase and, like all new technologies, has been met with skepticism, some deserved and some not, as we have seen through the evaluation of the data. There are clearly some limitations with the devices that are currently FDA approved. Presently, if you look at the value proposition of adopting robotic TKA, many studies have shown an increased cost through the capital purchase and through per case costs, for example, disposables.[6,15] In addition, all the studies have identified a learning curve where additional time is required to complete the TKA.[13,14,22,25–27] Although both of these factors diminish the cost-effectiveness of the technology, they seem to be self-limited, and become less significant once usage of the technology and the experience of the surgical team increases. Interestingly, however, none of the systems showed a decrease in quality during the learning curve. That is, clinical alignment was better than manual instruments and complications did not increase.

There is ample evidence to support the use of our present robotic systems for TKA during this introductory phase, given the clinical benefits that this technology offers for our patients today. However, if the adoption of robots continues on its present trajectory and surgical robots evolve like they have in other industries, it is expected that the future will hold many improvements. Looking forward, we can expect all robotic systems for TKA to offer robust preplanning coupled with the ability to adjust the plan dynamically to balance the soft tissue structures around the knee. All systems will be active, and the cutting tools will be efficient and offer haptic protection of the surrounding soft tissues.

From the perspective of the surgeon and the surgical support staff, implementation of robotic technology within the operating room should be easy and intuitive. Improvements will be made in human ergonomic usage of robots and ideally would allow full surgeon control within the sterile field. The graphic user interface should be plainly visible and easily manipulated within the surgical field: an active heads-up display. The robotic cutting tool should be as quiet as possible to minimize hearing loss in operating room participants. Advances in the workflow of future systems will maximize the productivity of the surgical team and minimize fatigue.

Finally, robot manufacturers and orthopedic device companies will support extensive training in the proper and efficient use of their robots to help launch successful surgeons to help optimize patient care. The robotic systems themselves will collect extensive data on the procedures themselves; for example, registration accuracy, joint dynamics, cut times and temperatures, bone quality, and robotic arm positions. All these data will be readily available to the surgeon, research personnel and developers of the technology itself. Artificial intelligence will be applied to mine these data to improve and refine algorithms for surgical preplanning and joint balancing to help us provide the best outcomes possible for our TKA patients.

CLINICS CARE POINTS

- Robotic assistance in TKA is still in its introductory phase and, like all new technologies, has been met with skepticism. The increased cost and duration of many robotic procedures, combined with a learning curve, all diminish the cost-effectiveness of this technology.

- Compared with manually instrumented TKA, robotic systems provide improved radiographic alignment and increased accuracy of component placement in concurrence with the surgical plan.

- Few systems assess the laxity of the final prosthetic joint in a standardized fashion by measuring the kinematic response of the joint under physiologic loading. Significant advancements are awaited connecting component positioning and joint laxity to improved outcomes and longevity.

- In the years ahead, all TKA robotic systems are expected to offer robust preoperative planning, coupled with the ability to adjust the plan dynamically to balance the soft tissue structures around the knee.

REFERENCES

1. Jacofsky DJ, Allen M. Robotics in arthroplasty: a comprehensive review. J Arthroplasty 2016;31: 2353–63.
2. Netravali NA, Shen F, Park Y, et al. A perspective on robotic assistance for knee arthroplasty. Adv Orthop 2013;2013:970703.
3. Song EK, Seon JK, Park SJ, et al. Simultaneous bilateral total knee arthroplasty with robotic and conventional techniques: a prospective, randomized study. Knee Surg Sports Traumatol Arthrosc 2011;19:1069–76.
4. Agarwal N, To K, McDonnell S, et al. Clinical and radiological outcomes in robotic-assisted total knee arthroplasty: a systematic review and meta-analysis. J Arthroplasty 2020;35(11):3393–409.e2.
5. Kayani B, Haddad FS. Robotic total knee arthroplasty: clinical outcomes and directions for future research. Bone Joint Res 2019;8:438–42.
6. Kayani B, Konan S, Ayuob A, et al. Robotic technology in total knee arthroplasty: a systematic review. EFORT Open Rev 2019;4:611–7.
7. Mont MA, Khlopas A, Chughtai M, et al. Value proposition of robotic total knee arthroplasty: what can robotic technology deliver in 2018 and beyond? Expert Rev Med Devices 2018;15:619–30.
8. Marchand RC, Sodhi N, Khlopas A, et al. Patient satisfaction outcomes after robotic arm-assisted total knee arthroplasty: a short-term evaluation. J Knee Surg 2017;30:849–53.
9. Khlopas A, Sodhi N, Hozack WJ, et al. Patient-reported functional and satisfaction outcomes after robotic-arm-assisted total knee arthroplasty: early results of a prospective multicenter investigation. J Knee Surg 2019;33(7):685–90.
10. Marchand RC, Khlopas A, Sodhi N, et al. Difficult cases in robotic arm-assisted total knee arthroplasty: a case series. J Knee Surg 2018;31:27–37.
11. Sultan AA, Samuel LT, Khlopas A, et al. Robotic-arm assisted total knee arthroplasty more accurately restored the posterior condylar offset ratio and the insall-salvati index compared to the manual technique; a cohort-matched study. Surg Technol Int 2019;34:409–13.
12. Hampp EL, Chughtai M, Scholl LY, et al. Robotic-arm assisted total knee arthroplasty demonstrated greater accuracy and precision to plan compared with manual techniques. J Knee Surg 2019;32: 239–50.
13. Sodhi N, Khlopas A, Piuzzi NS, et al. The learning curve associated with robotic total knee arthroplasty. J Knee Surg 2018;31:17–21.
14. Kayani B, Konan S, Huq SS, et al. Robotic-arm assisted total knee arthroplasty has a learning curve of seven cases for integration into the surgical workflow but no learning curve effect for accuracy of implant positioning. Knee Surg Sports Traumatol Arthrosc 2019;27:1132–41.
15. Moschetti WE, Konopka JF, Rubash HE, et al. Can robot-assisted unicompartmental knee arthroplasty be cost-effective? a Markov Decision Analysis. J Arthroplasty 2016;31:759–65.
16. Cool CL, Jacofsky DJ, Seeger KA, et al. A 90-day episode-of-care cost analysis of robotic-arm assisted total knee arthroplasty. J Comp Eff Res 2019; 8:327–36.
17. Stindel E, Briard JL, Merloz P, et al. Bone morphing: 3D morphological data for total knee arthroplasty. Comput Aided Surg 2002;7:156–68.
18. Lu TW, Chen HL, Chen SC. Comparisons of the lower limb kinematics between young and older adults when crossing obstacles of different heights. Gait Posture 2006;23:471–9.
19. König JA, Plaskos C. Improving value in TKA with robotics – evaluation of clinical and economic results with the OMNIBotics system. In: Lonner JH, editor. Robotics in knee and hip arthroplasty: current concepts, techniques and emerging uses. New York City: Springer; 2019. p. 172–9.
20. Suero EM, Plaskos C, Dixon PL, et al. Adjustable cutting blocks improve alignment and surgical time in computer-assisted total knee replacement. Knee Surg Sports Traumatol Arthrosc 2012;20: 1736–41.
21. Koulalis D, O'Loughlin PF, Plaskos C, et al. Sequential versus automated cutting guides in computer-assisted total knee arthroplasty. Knee 2011;18: 436–42.
22. Koenig JA, Suero EM, Plaskos C. Surgical accuracy and efficiency of computer-navigated TKA with a robotic cutting guide- Report on the first 100 cases. Orthop Proc 2012;94-B:103.
23. Ponder CE, Plaskos C, Cheal EJ. Press-fit total knee arthroplasty with a robotic-cutting guide: Proof of concept and initial clinical experience. Orthopaedic Proc 2013;95-B:61.
24. Koenig JA, Shalhoub S, Chen EA, et al. Accuracy of soft tissue balancing in robotic-assisted measured-resection TKA using a robotic distraction tool. In: Meere P, Baena FRY, editors. Accuracy of soft tissue balancing in robotic-assisted measured-resection TKA using a robotic distraction tool. New York City: EPiC Series in Health Sciences; 2019. p. 210–4.
25. Revenga C. 2015. Robotics and navigation. 2-year follow-up in navigated TKR. Results of a multicentre study. 16th EFORT Annual Congress. Prague, Czech Republic, 27 May 2015 - 29 May 2015.
26. Revenga C. 2016. 2-year follow-up of iBlock: robotic assisted surgery versus navigation in total knee arthroplasty. Results of a multicenter study. 17th EFORT Annual Congress. Geneva, Switzerland, 01 June 2016 - 03 June 2016.

27. Hernández-Vaquero D, Fernández-Carreira J, Revenga-Giertych C, et al. The use of PS or CR models is not sufficient to explain the differences in the results of total knee arthroplasty. study of interactions. J Adv Med Med Res 2015;12:1–9.

28. Keggi JM, Plaskos C. Learning curve and early patient satisfaction of robotic assisted total knee arthroplasty. Boston: International Society for Technology in Arthroplasty; 2016.

29. Keggi JM, Plaskos C. 2016. Surgical efficiency and early patient satisfaction in imageless robotic-assisted total knee arthroplasty. International Congress for Joint Reconstruction Transatlantic Orthopaedic Conference. New York City, NY, October 6-9, 2016.

30. Licini DJ, Meneghini RM. Modern abbreviated computer navigation of the femur reduces blood loss in total knee arthroplasty. J Arthroplasty 2015;30:1729–32.

31. Casper M, Mitra R, Khare R, et al. Accuracy assessment of a novel image-free handheld robot for Total Knee Arthroplasty in a cadaveric study. Comput Assist Surg (Abingdon) 2018;23:14–20.

32. Jaramaz B, Mitra R, Nikou C, et al. Technique and accuracy assessment of a novel image-free handheld robot for knee arthroplasty in bi-cruciate retaining total knee replacement. EPiC Ser Health Sci 2018;2:98–101.

33. Gregori A, Picard F, Lonner J, et al. 2015. Accuracy of imageless robotically assisted unicondylar knee arthroplasty. International Society for Computer Assisted Orthopaedic Surgery. Vancouver, Canada June 17-20, 2015.

34. Parratte S, Price AJ, Jeys LM, et al. Accuracy of a new robotically assisted technique for total knee arthroplasty: a cadaveric study. J Arthroplasty 2019;34:2799–803.

35. Seidenstein A, Birmingham M, Foran J, et al. Better accuracy and reproducibility of a new robotically-assisted system for total knee arthroplasty compared to conventional instrumentation: a cadaveric study. Knee Surg Sports Traumatol Arthrosc 2020. https://doi.org/10.1007/s00167-020-06038-w.

36. Bargar WL. Robots in orthopaedic surgery: past, present, and future. Clin Orthop Relat Res 2007;463:31–6.

37. Börner M, Wiesel U, Ditzen W. Clinical experiences with ROBODOC and the duracon total knee. navigation and robotics in total joint and spine surgery. Berlin: Springer Berlin Heidelberg; 2004. p. 362–6.

38. Liow MH, Chin PL, Tay KJ, et al. Early experiences with robot-assisted total knee arthroplasty using the DigiMatch ROBODOC(R) surgical system. Singapore Med J 2014;55:529–34.

39. Park SE, Lee CT. Comparison of robotic-assisted and conventional manual implantation of a primary total knee arthroplasty. J Arthroplasty 2007;22:1054–9.

40. Yang HY, Seon JK, Shin YJ, et al. Robotic total knee arthroplasty with a cruciate-retaining implant: a 10-year follow-up study. Clin Orthop Surg 2017;9:169–76.

41. Kim YH, Yoon SH, Park JW. Does robotic-assisted TKA result in better outcome scores or long-term survivorship than conventional TKA? A randomized, controlled trial. Clin orthopaedics Relat Res 2020;478:266–75.

42. Cho KJ, Seon JK, Jang WY, et al. Robotic versus conventional primary total knee arthroplasty: clinical and radiological long-term results with a minimum follow-up of ten years. Int Orthop 2019;43:1345–54.

43. Liow MHL, Goh GS, Wong MK, et al. Robotic-assisted total knee arthroplasty may lead to improvement in quality-of-life measures: a 2-year follow-up of a prospective randomized trial. Knee Surg Sports Traumatol Arthrosc 2017;25:2942–51.

44. Schache AG, Blanch P, Rath D, et al. Differences between the sexes in the three-dimensional angular rotations of the lumbo-pelvic-hip complex during treadmill running. J Sports Sci 2003;21:105–18.

Clinical Evidence of Current Irrigation Practices and the Use of Oral Antibiotics to Prevent and Treat Periprosthetic Joint Infection

Jason Zlotnicki, MD, Alexandra Grabrielli, MD,
Kenneth L. Urish, MD, PhD, Kimberly M. Brothers, PhD*

KEYWORDS

- Periprosthetic joint infection • Biofilm • Antibiotic • Lavage • Debridement

KEY POINTS

- Periprosthetic joint infection (PJI) is difficult to treat and a costly complication following total joint arthroplasty.
- Strategies aimed at reduction of PJI have great significance in the current health environment.
- Biofilm has a high tolerance to antibiotics, and this tolerance is induced by oxidative stress.

INTRODUCTION

During total joint arthroplasty, the contamination of the operative field with bacteria has historically been thought to be the major cause of early, acute periprosthetic joint infection (PJI).[1] Aimed at reducing this bacterial load, surgeons have engaged in the use of irrigation and other adjuvants during surgery and before wound closure. These additives have varied in type, concentration, and mechanism for disrupting bacterial colonization. Antiseptics, antibiotic-infused irrigation, or soap-like surfactants are three main classifications for irrigation solutions.[2] Oral antibiotics in the perioperative and postoperative period have been explored, whereas new advances continue to emerge for the prevention and treatment of acute PJI. This review examines some of the most widely reported interventions: dilute betadine/povidone-iodine, chlorhexidine, and hydrogen peroxide as lavage additives. Techniques for irrigation and extended oral antibiotic regimens are presented. The role of irrigants in PJI for treatment of planktonic and biofilm bacteria is discussed. Lastly, the newest advances in adjuvants for prevention of PJI are presented.

BETADINE/POVIDONE-IODINE

Dilute betadine lavage has been demonstrated in the literature to decrease rates of postoperative infection in orthopedic, urologic, cardiovascular, and general surgery procedures.[3,4] This is caused by the povidone-iodine contained within betadine, which releases free iodine in solution that is toxic to environmental microorganisms.[5] The success of this technique was first widely demonstrated in total joint arthroplasty by Brown and colleagues,[6] in which the occurrence of PJI in the first 90 postoperative days was reduced from 0.97% to 0.15% ($P = .04$). Additional

---

Arthritis and Arthroplasty Design Group, Department of Orthopaedic Surgery, College of Medicine, University of Pittsburgh, Bridgeside Point II, 450 Technology Drive, Pittsburgh, PA 15219, USA
* Corresponding author. Arthritis and Arthroplasty Design Group, Department of Orthopaedic Surgery, University of Pittsburgh Medical School, University of Pittsburgh, Bridgeside Point II, 450 Technology Drive, Pittsburgh, PA, 15219;
E-mail address: kmb227@pitt.edu

Orthop Clin N Am 52 (2021) 93–101
https://doi.org/10.1016/j.ocl.2020.12.002
0030-5898/21/© 2020 Elsevier Inc. All rights reserved.

advantages included that it was inexpensive, simple, and readily available within most operating rooms. Although larger reviews of the clinical studies have questioned the utility of this intervention,[7] further recent studies continue to demonstrate a potential role for dilute betadine irrigation in primary and revision arthroplasty.[8] A most recent randomized control clinical study comparing a 3-minute dilute betadine lavage with normal saline demonstrated a significant decrease in infection incidence (3.4% vs 0.4%; $P = .38$).[9] In the treatment of higher-risk PJI patients, dilute betadine has been demonstrated to be safe in combination with other substances including the antibiotic vancomycin.[10] Although a role for further cocktails may have utility, dilute betadine solution remains a possible option.

CHLORHEXIDINE

Chlorhexidine products have also started to receive attention as a potential intraoperative irrigant for the reduction of bacterial contamination. Historically studied and used as preoperative skin disinfectant, 2% chlorhexidine gluconate demonstrated a significant reduction in deep surgical site infections in multiple studies.[11,12] This is caused by chlorhexidine existing in cation form at physiologic pH, allowing it to bind to negatively charged bacterial membranes; this leads to bacteriostatic and bactericidal effects at low and high concentrations, respectively.[13] Despite the excellent data with preoperative skin cleansing, the data for intraoperative use have been inconsistent. A study by Frisch and colleagues[14] did not detect any difference in infection reduction at 1 year with the use of chlorhexidine gluconate when comparing with dilute povidone-iodine and saline. In the case of a known infection, in vitro studies have shown a significant decrease in bacterial colony-forming units of biofilm forming staphylococcal species.[15] However, larger clinical studies are needed to detect a benefit for the use of chlorhexidine for the prevention and treatment of PJI. Older studies have demonstrated success with a combination of chlorhexidine and hydrogen peroxide,[16] with theoretic benefit of a kill of a wider range of organisms with lower concentrations of each substance.

HYDROGEN PEROXIDE

As cases of complex infection and resistant species arise, more aggressive debridement strategies are being tested for the treatment of colonized joints.[17] This includes the use of hydrogen peroxide, which despite decades of use in wound treatment has only recently emerged in the treatment of total joint arthroplasty. Historically, hydrogen peroxide has been demonstrated to be widely effective in vivo in killing bacteria, through numerous pathways, including oxidative stress.[18–20] Clinical studies have demonstrated mixed results across multiple surgical specialties, especially when used in isolation.[21–23] Recent studies in total joint arthroplasty have demonstrated more success when used in combination with other antimicrobial irrigation fluids, specifically povidone-iodine. George and colleagues[24] demonstrated excellent clinical outcomes in prevention of infection recurrence in 39 total joint arthroplasties, at a mean of 6 years after single-stage exchange arthroplasty, using a combination of povidone-iodine and diluted hydrogen peroxide. However, the complications of cytotoxicity and air embolism associated with the effervescence have been documented in the literature, with some suggesting no role for peroxide in orthopaedic surgical care.[25,26]

Overall, there are several clinical studies with variable results at adding povidone-iodine, chlorhexidine, or hydrogen peroxide to irrigants to prevent PJI. An important observation is the absence of clinical studies at using these adjuvants in the treatment of PJI. The use of bactericidal compounds seems to be logical in the treatment of PJI, but appreciating that oxidative stress can induce biofilm antibiotic tolerance (discussed later) may create a more complicated picture.

PULSE LAVAGE VERSUS GRAVITY IRRIGATION

Aside from adding antimicrobials and surfactants to irrigation fluid, study has been directed at the effect of irrigation delivery into the surgical wound bed. The American College of Surgeons has classified irrigation method as either high (ie, pulsed lavage system) or low pressure (ie, bulb syringe, gravity flow).[27] An early study examining Staphylococcus aureus inoculation removal in vitro demonstrated that high and low pressure were equivalent at early time points, but low-pressure irrigation no longer had effect after 6 hours.[28] Although further studies demonstrated superiority of higher pressure irrigation,[29] additional study demonstrated higher levels of tissue damage, larger bacterial burden rebound, and the propagation of bacteria into deep tissues.[30–32] Most recently, the Fluid Lavage of Open Wounds (FLOW) study, conducted in the investigation of open fractures, has shown no difference in reoperation rates between low- and high-pressure systems.[28] Therefore, although high-pressure systems may be more effective in decreasing bacterial counts, injury to local soft tissues and bacterial rebound must be taken into account in the care of surgical wound beds. Ultimately, the best available current evidence suggests that there is no difference between these two methods.

ORAL ANTIBIOTICS FOR PROPHYLAXIS AND TREATMENT

In addition to the use of adjuvant irrigation techniques for high-risk patients or known cases of PJI, the use of an extended postoperative oral antibiotic regimen has been theorized to provide benefit. In a study examining patients deemed high risk for PJI on basis of specific risk factors, high-risk patients who did not receive a 7-day course of oral antibiotic on discharge were more than four times more likely to develop PJI.[33] In this study, patients received cefadroxil, 500 mg twice a day, unless they tested positive for methicillin-resistant S. aureus (MRSA) in preoperative assessment mandating the use of sulfamethoxazole-trimethoprim DS twice a day. If they had documented anaphylaxis to cephalosporins, they were given 300 mg of clindamycin three times a day.[33] In settings of known PJI, debridement and antibiotics with implant retention (DAIR) and two-stage exchange are the most common techniques used. Following the irrigation and debridement, systemic antibiotics are used for approximately 6 weeks, although Infectious Diseases Society of America guidelines allow for a range in treatment. Based on the high failure rate, almost 60%,[34] associated with DAIR procedures, the use of oral antibiotics for an undisclosed length of time has become increasingly popular. A recent large clinical study of DAIR procedures has strong evidence that extended use of oral antibiotics for 1 year can decrease failure rates, was not associated with increased adverse events, and provided guidelines for antibiotic stewardship, because treatment was only required for a defined time period.[35] The other common treatment of PJI includes two-stage exchange arthroplasty with reported success rates ranging from 67% to 91% depending on the definition of success.[36] However, this leaves significant room for improvement in the eradication of infection and successful implant survival at later time points after two-stage. A recent multicenter randomized study examining a 3-month course of oral antibiotics against no antibiotics demonstrated that the treatment group failed two-stage revision less frequently than those not receiving antibiotics (5% vs 19%; P = .016).[37] These findings are further supported by a more recent randomized controlled trial demonstrating reduction of infection recurrence rate after a 3-month oral course following two-stage revision, 12.5% (antibiotics) versus 28.6% (no antibiotics).[38] Other groups have demonstrated the valuable role of tranexamic acid in reducing the rates of PJI, likely through decreasing the presence of a postoperative hematoma.[39] This highlights the need for continued study of postoperative organism-directed antibiotic therapy, in addition to intraoperative strategies.

BIOFILM ANTIBIOTIC TOLERANCE

Irrigation and debridement are the gold standard for management and treatment of PJI. However, this treatment fails in 60% of cases.[40] As bacteria multiply in infections they transition from the free-swimming or the planktonic form and cluster together to form large aggregates composed of an extracellular matrix called a biofilm. A biofilm can contain 1000 to 10,000 times more bacteria growing than in the planktonic form.[41] In comparison with their planktonic counterparts, biofilms are as much as 1000 times more resistant to biocides.[41,42] The biofilm extracellular matrix is largely responsible for this resistance. The biofilm extracellular matrix consists of polysaccharides, nucleic acids, and protein, all of which are believed to contribute to antibiotic tolerance.[42–44] Mandell and colleagues demonstrated the minimum inhibitory concentration and the minimum bactericidal concentration were much higher in biofilms in comparison to planktonic bacteria in PJI clinical isolates of S. aureus.[42,43,45] Similarly, Koch and colleagues[46] demonstrated similar findings in PJI clinical isolates of Staphylococcus epidermidis and Cutibacterium acnes. Antibiotic tolerance in PJI is believed to occur through (1) the development of bacterial persister cells[47] that are able to survive in the presence of antibiotics,[48] (2) an overall decreased bacterial metabolism when in the biofilm state,[49] and (3) the thick extracellular polymeric substance that binds and prevents drug penetration into the biofilm.[43,50]

PERSISTER CELLS AND TOXIN-ANTITOXIN SYSTEMS

Persister cells[47] are a small population of bacteria that are highly tolerant to antibiotics without undergoing any genetic changes.[51] It is hypothesized that they are less sensitive to antibiotics because their cellular metabolism is dormant and thus not susceptible to antibiotic targets. Their antibiotic tolerance in the biofilm state is accomplished through toxin-antitoxin systems. This system is composed of a toxin that is able to disrupt an important cellular process and an antitoxin that prevents toxin activation. The toxin and antitoxin form a complex in conditions of normal homeostasis. When the bacterium encounters an environmental stress (ie, antibiotic treatment), the antitoxin disassembles from the toxin. The toxin becomes activated and disrupts bacterial metabolism to induce a state of dormancy.[48,52,53] This system allows the bacteria to become tolerant to antibiotics. When treatment is stopped, the antitoxin binds to the toxin resuming metabolic activities and antibiotic sensitivity. Toxin-antitoxin systems have been well studied in gram-negative bacteria. In *Escherichia coli* toxin-antitoxin systems were identified to play a role in persistence and antibiotic tolerance.[54] In *Mycobacterium tuberculosis* toxin-antitoxin systems were shown to play a role in antibiotic tolerance, environmental stress adaptation, and virulence.[55] In studies by Ma and colleagues the *S. aureus* toxin-antitoxin system *MazEF* was demonstrated to play a role in biofilm formation, antibiotic tolerance, and infection.[56]

OXIDATIVE STRESS AGENTS AND BIOFILM ANTIBIOTIC TOLERANCE

Many studies have demonstrated the positive benefit of oxidative stress-inducing agents in removal of biofilms. Schwecter and colleagues[57] demonstrated disruption of MRSA biofilms with chlorhexidine gluconate. Lineback and colleagues[58] found hydrogen peroxide and sodium hypochlorite were more effective against *S. aureus* and *Pseudomonas aeruginosa* biofilms than quaternary ammonium compounds. However, given what has been previously discussed on effective irrigation solutions and biofilm antibiotic tolerance, oxidative stress-inducing agents, such as hydrogen peroxide, povidone-iodine, and chlorhexidine, have also been demonstrated to inhibit bacterial metabolism[49] thus increasing their tolerance to antibiotics.

Several studies have demonstrated the ability of these agents to be effective against planktonic bacteria but fail to significantly reduce the bacterial burden of biofilm bacteria.[59] Rowe and colleagues[60] demonstrated oxidative stress agents halt bacterial metabolism and induce persistence

in *S. aureus* planktonic cells. In addition, several studies have demonstrated biofilm resistance to hydrogen peroxide.[61–63] Elkins and colleagues[62] found two catalases provided protection to *P. aeruginosa* biofilms when exposed to hydrogen peroxide. Hydrogen peroxide enhanced biofilm formation in a mucoid *P. aeruginosa* strain by promoting overproduction of alginate, a component of its extracellular matrix in a study by Tan and colleagues.[64] Leung and colleagues[63] found after a 5-minute exposure of biofilms to clinically relevant concentrations of hydrogen peroxide, most *Candida albicans* and *E. coli* biofilms were intact and alive. Tote and colleagues[65] focused on several biocides and their ability to remove planktonic and biofilm bacteria. As expected most biocides could eliminate planktonic bacteria but failed to eliminate the biofilm. Povidone-iodine and hydrogen peroxide were effective enough with a 5 log reduction of planktonic *P. aeruginosa* after a 5-minute contact time. After treatment with povidone-iodine and hydrogen peroxide a 5 log reduction was observed in *S. aureus* planktonic growth after 5 and 15 minutes, respectively. Of all the biocides tested in this study, sodium hypochlorite and hydrogen peroxide had the greatest activity on *P. aeruginosa* and *S. aureus* biofilms because of their ability to target the biofilm biomass and the extracellular matrix. Hydrogen peroxide was able to reduce *S. aureus* biofilms by 89% after only 1 minute. This efficacy was not as rapid for *P. aeruginosa* but did result in complete eradication of biofilms after 60 minutes of treatment. Povidone-iodine had a greater efficacy and reduced *P. aeruginosa* biofilms by 94% after only a 1-minute contact time. Chlorhexidine digluconate was far more effective at targeting *S. aureus* resulting in an 84% decrease in viability after a 1-minute contact time in comparison with a 40% reduction in viability of *P. aeruginosa* biofilms. These differences in microbicidal activity are most likely caused by the composition of the bacterial cell walls because *S. aureus* is a gram-positive bacterium and *P. aeruginosa* is gram-negative. Hardy and colleagues[66] cautioned repeated exposure of *S. aureus* to biocides. Significant increases in antibiotic minimum inhibitory concentrations and minimum bactericidal concentrations were observed after repeated exposures of clinical isolates to chlorhexidine.

THE IMPACT OF MOVING FLUIDS ON BIOFILM PHYSIOLOGY

Many groups have focused on how the movement of fluids impacts biofilm formation. Biofilms have been described as viscoelastic.[67]

Work by Böl and colleagues and Blauert and colleagues has demonstrated under certain conditions the same biofilm can behave as a fluid, a solid, or a mixture of the two.[68,69] Flow cell experiments where growth media is flowed directly across a growing biofilm have shown that biofilms are able to rearrange their macroscopic structure in response to shear stressing forces to form more "drag-like" forms, such as streamers or ripples.[70] Biofilms with ripple or wavy patterns have been found growing inside endotracheal tubes[71] and venous catheters.[72] In an elegant study by Fabbri and colleagues[73] the rippling effect of the biofilm was studied using a compressed air jet. Ripple-like structures were observed to form at the biofilm/fluid interface in *Streptococcus mutans* and *S. epidermidis*. A wrinkly phenotype was observed to form rapidly in *P. aeruginosa* biofilms and was more resistant to disturbance by the air jet. The authors hypothesized these differences in biofilm phenotypes were likely caused by differences in the extracellular matrix that formed each biofilm. These studies highlight how the extracellular matrix of the biofilm can allow it to survive elimination attempts, such as irrigation in the context of orthopedic infections.

As previously discussed, high-pressure systems may be more effective in decreasing bacterial burden. The role of high-pressure (pulse lavage) irrigation in biofilm clearance was explored by Urish and colleagues.[74] *S. aureus* biofilms were grown on three different total knee arthroplasty materials: cobalt chrome metal, polymethyl methacrylate, and polyethylene. The biofilm biomass was quantified before and after pulse lavage irrigation. The biofilm was nearly eradicated from cobalt chrome metal, but polymethyl methacrylate and polyethylene only had a 10-fold reduction in biomass. These results indicate even after pulse lavage irrigation a significant amount of the biofilm remains on the implant surface. These results indicate under these circumstances antibiotic treatment would be unlikely to effectively eliminate infection.

AUGMENTING CURRENT THERAPIES AND UPCOMING TECHNOLOGIES

In addition to organism-directed antibiotic antibiotics, therapies that can effectively eradicate biofilms are also necessary. Biofilms continue to be a problem because of their action as a barrier against mechanical debridement, antibiotics administration, and the effects of the host's immune system. Treatment strategies surrounding biofilm infections involve optimizing and augmenting current treatment algorithms and investigating novel avenues that might aid in the eradication of biofilms. It has been established that rifampin may be an adjunct to use with other antibiotics for the treatment of PJI.[75,76] Greimel and colleagues[77] explored possible synergistic activities of rifampin combined with moxifloxacin using a mouse model of PJI. This study exhibited that the combination therapy has superior bactericidal effects compared with the monotherapy after 14 days of treatment.[77] Beyond antibiotic adjuvants, additional novel therapies are being investigated. Specific nanoparticles are beginning to be identified as having passive antibiotic properties that could be beneficial in the treatment of PJI. Certain nanoparticles are able to lyse bacterial cells by increasing the concentrations of reactive oxygen species and decreased the integrity of the cell membrane and wall. Zaidi and colleagues[78] demonstrated that some inorganic nanoparticles (zinc oxide, silver, copper) have bactericidal modes of action and would be challenging for bacteria to develop resistance to. A rat model for MRSA wound infection showed faster wound healing and formation of collagen fibers using nanoparticles.[79] This technology has yet to be tested in an in vivo PJI model but does show promise. Mandell and colleagues[80,81] demonstrate a cationic antimicrobial peptide WLBU2 can effectively eliminate methicillin-sensitive *S. aureus* and MRSA clinical isolate biofilms. This peptide was still effective in the presence of bacteria with inhibited metabolism suggesting a promising future for its use as an antimicrobial therapy.[80]

SUMMARY

In periprosthetic infection, dilute betadine, chlorhexidine, and hydrogen peroxide have been shown to be effective against treatment of planktonic bacteria. However, this treatment largely fails because of the presence of antibiotic-tolerant biofilm. Repeated exposure to oxidative stress-inducing biocides in irrigant solutions and reduced bacterial metabolism in the biofilm state contribute to this antibiotic tolerance. The use of antiseptics as irrigants should be carefully considered and only used when deemed necessary. Future studies focused on combination therapies of these antiseptics and eradication of biofilms should be explored.

CLINICS CARE POINTS

- The use of dilute betadine or chlorhexidine solution as an additive to irrigation solution may prevent PJI, but further study is needed.
- Because of its mixed results for efficacy, the use of hydrogen peroxide as an irrigant requires further study.
- Both high- (pulsed lavage systems) or low-pressure irrigation are equivalent resulting in a reduction in biofilm mass.
- Oral antibiotics may prevent PJI in high-risk patients following arthroplasty surgery and improve treatment outcomes in DAIR and two-stage exchanges.
- Biofilms are highly antibiotic tolerant.
- Antibiotic tolerance is mediated by toxin-antitoxin systems.
- Reduced bacterial metabolism contributes to antibiotic tolerance.
- Biofilms are largely resistant to forces applied to their outer surface limiting the effectiveness of irrigation and debridement.
- Combination therapies with irrigants and alternative strategies are necessary to eradicate biofilms in PJI.

DISCLOSURE

This work was support by grant number K08AR071494 to KLU.

REFERENCES

1. Charnley J. Postoperative infection after total hip replacement with special reference to air contamination in the operating room. Clin Orthop Relat Res 1972;87:167–87.
2. Ruder JA, Springer BD. Treatment of periprosthetic joint infection using antimicrobials: dilute povidone-iodine lavage. J Bone Jt Infect 2017; 2(1):10–4.
3. Chundamala J, Wright JG. The efficacy and risks of using povidone-iodine irrigation to prevent surgical site infection: an evidence-based review. Can J Surg 2007;50(6):473–81.
4. Cheng MT, Chang MC, Wang ST, et al. Efficacy of dilute betadine solution irrigation in the prevention of postoperative infection of spinal surgery. Spine 1976;30(15):1689–93.
5. Oduwole KO, Glynn AA, Molony DC, et al. Anti-biofilm activity of sub-inhibitory povidone-iodine

concentrations against Staphylococcus epidermidis and Staphylococcus aureus. J Orthop Res 2010; 28(9):1252–6.
6. Brown NM, Cipriano CA, Moric M, et al. Dilute betadine lavage before closure for the prevention of acute postoperative deep periprosthetic joint infection. J Arthroplasty 2012;27(1):27–30.
7. Hernandez NM, Hart A, Taunton MJ, et al. Use of povidone-iodine irrigation prior to wound closure in primary total hip and knee arthroplasty: an analysis of 11,738 cases. J Bone Joint Surg Am 2019; 101(13):1144–50.
8. Slullitel PA, Dobransky JS, Bali K, et al. Is there a role for preclosure dilute betadine irrigation in the prevention of postoperative infection following total joint arthroplasty? J Arthroplasty 2020;35(5):1374–8.
9. Calkins TE, Culvern C, Nam D, et al. Dilute betadine lavage reduces the risk of acute postoperative periprosthetic joint infection in aseptic revision total knee and hip arthroplasty: a randomized controlled trial. J Arthroplasty 2020;35(2):538.e1.
10. Iorio R, Yu S, Anoushiravani AA, et al. Vancomycin powder and dilute povidone-iodine lavage for infection prophylaxis in high-risk total joint arthroplasty. J Arthroplasty 2020;35(7):1933–6.
11. Kapadia BH, Johnson AJ, Daley JA, et al. Pre-admission cutaneous chlorhexidine preparation reduces surgical site infections in total hip arthroplasty. J Arthroplasty 2013;28(3):490–3.
12. Zywiel MG, Daley JA, Delanois RE, et al. Advance pre-operative chlorhexidine reduces the incidence of surgical site infections in knee arthroplasty. Int Orthop 2011;35(7):1001–6.
13. Milstone AM, Passaretti CL, Perl TM. Chlorhexidine: expanding the armamentarium for infection control and prevention. Clin Infect Dis 2008;46(2):274–81.
14. Frisch NB, Kadri OM, Tenbrunsel T, et al. Intraoperative chlorhexidine irrigation to prevent infection in total hip and knee arthroplasty. Arthroplast Today 2017;3(4):294–7.
15. Smith DC, Maiman R, Schwechter EM, et al. Optimal irrigation and debridement of infected total joint implants with chlorhexidine gluconate. J Arthroplasty 2015;30(10):1820–2.
16. Steinberg D, Heling I, Daniel I, et al. Antibacterial synergistic effect of chlorhexidine and hydrogen peroxide against Streptococcus sobrinus, Streptococcus faecalis and Staphylococcus aureus. J Oral Rehabil 1999;26(2):151–6.
17. Lu M, Hansen EN. Hydrogen peroxide wound irrigation in orthopaedic surgery. J Bone Jt Infect 2017;2(1):3–9.
18. McDonnell G, Russell AD. Antiseptics and disinfectants: activity, action, and resistance. Clin Microbiol Rev 1999;12(1):147–79.
19. Brown CD, Zitelli JA. A review of topical agents for wounds and methods of wounding. Guidelines for

wound management. J Dermatol Surg Oncol 1993; 19(8):732–7.

20. Imlay JA, Chin SM, Linn S. Toxic DNA damage by hydrogen peroxide through the Fenton reaction in vivo and in vitro. Science 1988;240(4852):640–2.

21. Lau WY, Wong SH. Randomized, prospective trial of topical hydrogen peroxide in appendectomy wound infection. High risk factors. Am J Surg 1981;142(3):393–7.

22. Leyden JJ, Bartelt NM. Comparison of topical antibiotic ointments, a wound protectant, and antiseptics for the treatment of human blister wounds contaminated with Staphylococcus aureus. J Fam Pract 1987;24(6):601–4.

23. Mohammadi AA, Seyed Jafari SM, Kiasat M, et al. Efficacy of debridement and wound cleansing with 2% hydrogen peroxide on graft take in the chronic-colonized burn wounds; a randomized controlled clinical trial. Burns 2013;39(6):1131–6.

24. George DA, Konan S, Haddad FS. Single-stage hip and knee exchange for periprosthetic joint infection. J Arthroplasty 2015;30(12):2264–70.

25. DePaula CA, Truncale KG, Gertzman AA, et al. Effects of hydrogen peroxide cleaning procedures on bone graft osteoinductivity and mechanical properties. Cell Tissue Bank 2005;6(4):287–98.

26. Kleffmann J, Ferbert A, Deinsberger W, et al. Extensive ischemic brainstem lesions and pneumocephalus after application of hydrogen peroxide (H2O2) during lumbar spinal surgery. Spine J 2015;15(4):e5–7.

27. Souba WW. ACS surgery: principles and practice. 6th edition. New York: WebMD, Inc.; 2007.

28. Bhandari M, Schemitsch EH, Adili A, et al. High and low pressure pulsatile lavage of contaminated tibial fractures: an in vitro study of bacterial adherence and bone damage. J Orthop Trauma 1999;13(8):526–33.

29. Svoboda SJ, Bice TG, Gooden HA, et al. Comparison of bulb syringe and pulsed lavage irrigation with use of a bioluminescent musculoskeletal wound model. J Bone Joint Surg Am 2006;88(10):2167–74.

30. Owens BD, White DW, Wenke JC. Comparison of irrigation solutions and devices in a contaminated musculoskeletal wound survival model. J Bone Joint Surg Am 2009;91(1):92–8.

31. Boyd JI 3rd, Wongworawat MD. High-pressure pulsatile lavage causes soft tissue damage. Clin Orthop Relat Res 2004;427:13–7.

32. Hassinger SM, Harding G, Wongworawat MD. High-pressure pulsatile lavage propagates bacteria into soft tissue. Clin Orthop Relat Res 2005;439:27–31.

33. Inabathula A, Dilley JE, Ziemba-Davis M, et al. Extended oral antibiotic prophylaxis in high-risk patients substantially reduces primary total hip and knee arthroplasty 90-day infection rate. J Bone Joint Surg Am 2018;100(24):2103–9.

34. Urish KL, Bullock AG, Kreger AM, et al. A multicenter study of irrigation and debridement in total knee arthroplasty periprosthetic joint infection: treatment failure is high. J Arthroplasty 2018; 33(4):1154–9.

35. Shah NB, Hersh BL, Kreger A, et al. Benefits and adverse events associated with extended antibiotic use in total knee arthroplasty periprosthetic joint infection. Clin Infect Dis 2020;70:559–65.

36. Mortazavi SM, Vegari D, Ho A, et al. Two-stage exchange arthroplasty for infected total knee arthroplasty: predictors of failure. Clin Orthop Relat Res 2011;469(11):3049–54.

37. Frank JM, Kayupov E, Moric M, et al. The Mark Coventry, MD, Award: oral antibiotics reduce reinfection after two-stage exchange: a multicenter, randomized controlled trial. Clin Orthop Relat Res 2017;475(1):56–61.

38. Yang J, Parvizi J, Hansen EN, et al. 2020 Mark Coventry Award: microorganism-directed oral antibiotics reduce the rate of failure due to further infection after two-stage revision hip or knee arthroplasty for chronic infection: a multicentre randomized controlled trial at a minimum of two years. Bone Joint J 2020;102-B(6_Supple_A):3–9.

39. Drain NP, Gobao VC, Bertolini DM, et al. Administration of tranexamic acid improves long-term outcomes in total knee arthroplasty. J Arthroplasty 2020;35(6S):S201–6.

40. Angelini A, Drago G, Trovarelli G, et al. Infection after surgical resection for pelvic bone tumors: an analysis of 270 patients from one institution. Clin Orthop Relat Res 2014;472(1):349–59.

41. Costerton JW, Geesey GG, Cheng KJ. How bacteria stick. Sci Am 1978;238(1):86–95.

42. Ma D, Shanks RMQ, Davis CM, et al. Viable bacteria persist on antibiotic spacers following two-stage revision for periprosthetic joint infection. J Orthop Res 2018;36:452–8.

43. Urish KL, DeMuth PW, Kwan BW, et al. Antibiotic-tolerant Staphylococcus aureus biofilm persists on arthroplasty materials. Clin Orthop Relat Res 2016;474(7):1649–56.

44. Peel TN, Buising KL, Choong PF. Prosthetic joint infection: challenges of diagnosis and treatment. ANZ J Surg 2011;81(1–2):32–9.

45. Mandell JB, Orr S, Koch J, et al. Large variations in clinical antibiotic activity against Staphylococcus aureus biofilms of periprosthetic joint infection isolates. J Orthop Res 2019;37(7):1604–9.

46. Koch JA, Pust TM, Cappellini AJ, et al. Staphylococcus epidermidis biofilms have a high tolerance to antibiotics in periprosthetic joint infection. Life (Basel) 2020;10(11):253.

47. Balaban NQ, Helaine S, Lewis K, et al. Definitions and guidelines for research on antibiotic persistence. Nat Rev Microbiol 2019;17(7):441–8.

48. Kwan BW, Valenta JA, Benedik MJ, et al. Arrested protein synthesis increases persister-like cell formation. Antimicrob Agents Chemother 2013;57(3):1468–73.

49. Brindle ER, Miller DA, Stewart PS. Hydrodynamic deformation and removal of *Staphylococcus epidermidis* biofilms treated with urea, chlorhexidine, iron chloride, or DispersinB. Biotechnol Bioeng 2011;108(12):2968–77.

50. Neut D, van der Mei HC, Bulstra SK, et al. The role of small-colony variants in failure to diagnose and treat biofilm infections in orthopedics. Acta Orthop 2007;78(3):299–308.

51. Lewis K. Persister cells. Annu Rev Microbiol 2010; 64:357–72.

52. Wang X, Lord DM, Cheng HY, et al. A new type V toxin-antitoxin system where mRNA for toxin GhoT is cleaved by antitoxin GhoS. Nat Chem Biol 2012;8(10):855–61.

53. Fasani RA, Savageau MA. Molecular mechanisms of multiple toxin-antitoxin systems are coordinated to govern the persister phenotype. Proc Natl Acad Sci U S A 2013;110(27):E2528–37.

54. Tripathi A, Dewan PC, Siddique SA, et al. MazF-induced growth inhibition and persister generation in *Escherichia coli*. J Biol Chem 2014;289(7):4191–205.

55. Tiwari P, Arora G, Singh M, et al. MazF ribonucleases promote *Mycobacterium tuberculosis* drug tolerance and virulence in guinea pigs. Nat Commun 2015;6:6059.

56. Ma D, Mandell JB, Donegan NP, et al. The toxin-antitoxin MazEF drives *Staphylococcus aureus* biofilm formation, antibiotic tolerance, and chronic infection. mBio 2019;10(6). https://doi.org/10.1128/mBio.01658-19.

57. Schwechter EM, Folk D, Varshney AK, et al. Optimal irrigation and debridement of infected joint implants: an in vitro methicillin-resistant *Staphylococcus aureus* biofilm model. J Arthroplasty 2011; 26(6 Suppl):109–13.

58. Lineback CB, Nkemngong CA, Wu ST, et al. Hydrogen peroxide and sodium hypochlorite disinfectants are more effective against *Staphylococcus aureus* and *Pseudomonas aeruginosa* biofilms than quaternary ammonium compounds. Antimicrob Resist Infect Control 2018;7:154.

59. Smith K, Hunter IS. Efficacy of common hospital biocides with biofilms of multi-drug resistant clinical isolates. J Med Microbiol 2008;57(Pt 8):966–73.

60. Rowe SE, Wagner NJ, Li L, et al. Reactive oxygen species induce antibiotic tolerance during systemic *Staphylococcus aureus* infection. Nat Microbiol 2020;5(2):282–90.

61. Khakimova M, Ahlgren HG, Harrison JJ, et al. The stringent response controls catalases in *Pseudomonas aeruginosa* and is required for hydrogen peroxide and antibiotic tolerance. J Bacteriol 2013;195(9):2011–20.

62. Elkins JG, Hassett DJ, Stewart PS, et al. Protective role of catalase in *Pseudomonas aeruginosa* biofilm resistance to hydrogen peroxide. Appl Environ Microbiol 1999;65(10):4594–600.

63. Leung CY, Chan YC, Samaranayake LP, et al. Biocide resistance of *Candida* and *Escherichia coli* biofilms is associated with higher antioxidative capacities. J Hosp Infect 2012;81(2):79–86.

64. Tan Q, Ai Q, Xu Q, et al. Polymorphonuclear leukocytes or hydrogen peroxide enhance biofilm development of mucoid *Pseudomonas aeruginosa*. Mediators Inflamm 2018;2018:8151362. https://doi.org/10.1155/2018/8151362.

65. Tote K, Horemans T, Vanden Berghe D, et al. Inhibitory effect of biocides on the viable masses and matrices of *Staphylococcus aureus* and *Pseudomonas aeruginosa* biofilms. Appl Environ Microbiol 2010;76(10):3135–42.

66. Hardy K, Sunnucks K, Gil H, et al. Increased usage of antiseptics is associated with reduced susceptibility in clinical isolates of *Staphylococcus aureus*. mBio 2018;9(3). https://doi.org/10.1128/mBio.00894-18.

67. Stoodley P, Lewandowski Z, Boyle JD, et al. Structural deformation of bacterial biofilms caused by short-term fluctuations in fluid shear: an in situ investigation of biofilm rheology. Biotechnol Bioeng 1999;65(1):83–92.

68. Bol M, Möhle RB, Haesner M, et al. 3D finite element model of biofilm detachment using real biofilm structures from CLSM data. Biotechnol Bioeng 2009;103(1):177–86.

69. Blauert F, Horn H, Wagner M. Time-resolved biofilm deformation measurements using optical coherence tomography. Biotechnol Bioeng 2015; 112(9):1893–905.

70. Stoodley P, Lewandowski Z, Boyle JD, et al. The formation of migratory ripples in a mixed species bacterial biofilm growing in turbulent flow. Environ Microbiol 1999;1(5):447–55.

71. Inglis TJ. Evidence for dynamic phenomena in residual tracheal tube biofilm. Br J Anaesth 1993;70(1):22–4.

72. Rusconi R, Lecuyer S, Guglielmini L, et al. Laminar flow around corners triggers the formation of biofilm streamers. J R Soc Interf 2010; 7(50):1293–9.

73. Fabbri S, Li J, Howlin RP, et al. Fluid-driven interfacial instabilities and turbulence in bacterial biofilms. Environ Microbiol 2017;19(11):4417–31.

74. Urish KL, DeMuth PW, Craft DW, et al. Pulse lavage is inadequate at removal of biofilm from the surface of total knee arthroplasty materials. J Arthroplasty 2014;29(6):1128–32.

75. Zimmerli W, Widmer AF, Blatter M, et al. Role of rifampin for treatment of orthopedic implant-related staphylococcal infections: a randomized controlled trial. Foreign-Body Infection (FBI) Study Group. JAMA 1998;279(19):1537–41.

76. O'Reilly T, Kunz S, Sande E, et al. Relationship between antibiotic concentration in bone and efficacy of treatment of staphylococcal osteomyelitis in rats: azithromycin compared with clindamycin and rifampin. Antimicrob Agents Chemother 1992; 36(12):2693–7.

77. Greimel F, Scheuerer C, Gessner A, et al. Efficacy of antibiotic treatment of implant-associated *Staphylococcus aureus* infections with moxifloxacin, flucloxacillin, rifampin, and combination therapy: an animal study. Drug Des Devel Ther 2017;11:1729–36.

78. Zaidi S, Misba L, Khan AU. Nano-therapeutics: a revolution in infection control in post antibiotic era. Nanomedicine 2017;13(7):2281–301.

79. Li YJ, Harroun SG, Su YC, et al. Synthesis of self-assembled spermidine-carbon quantum dots effective against multidrug-resistant bacteria. Adv Healthc Mater 2016;5(19):2545–54.

80. Mandell JB, Deslouches B, Montelaro RC, et al. Elimination of antibiotic resistant surgical implant biofilms using an engineered cationic amphipathic peptide WLBU2. Sci Rep 2017;7(1). https://doi.org/10.1038/s41598-017-17780-6.

81. Mandell JB, Koch J, Deslouches B, et al. Direct antimicrobial activity of cationic amphipathic peptide WLBU2 against *Staphylococcus aureus* biofilms is enhanced in physiologic buffered saline. J Orthop Res 2020;38(12):2657.

Opioid Use Patterns After Primary Total Knee Replacement

Karen J. Derefinko, PhD[a],*, Zhenghua Gong, MS[b],
Zoran Bursac, PhD[b], Sarah B. Hand, MPH, CCRP[c],
Karen C. Johnson, MD, MPH[d],
William M. Mihalko, MD, PhD[e]

KEYWORDS

• Opioids • Total knee replacement • Controlled substance monitoring • Pain

KEY POINTS

- The authors examined controlled substance prescriptions following total knee replacement (TKR) surgery in a sample of 560 TKR patients.
- Results indicated that of all the 5164 prescriptions documented on the controlled substance monitoring database, 64% were for opioid medications.
- Over half of the patients received controlled substances from both the surgery site provider and a nonsurgery site provider in the year following surgery.
- The authors recommend that providers consider the possibility of outside prescribing when prescribing opioid analgesic.

INTRODUCTION

According to the 2017 National Survey on Drug Use and Health data, 11.4 million Americans over the age of 12 reported the misuse of opioid medication in the past year, demonstrating that opioid misuse is a critical public health problem.[1,2] Misuse is generally defined as an intentional therapeutic use of a drug in an inappropriate way.[3] Some forms of opioid misuse can have very severe consequences. For instance, the Centers for Disease Control and Prevention developed a flyer for prescribers that describes overdose risk categories.[4] This flyer indicates that even lower use (20–50 morphine milligram equivalents [MME] per day) increases risk of overdose, a finding supported by meta-analytic research,[5] and risk of overdose doubles when use is at or greater than 50 MMEs/d (vs <20 MMEs).

Funding: K.J. Derefinko, S.B. Hand, and K.C. Johnson were supported in part by the National Center for Complementary & Integrative Health of the National Institutes of Health under award number R61AT010604. The content is solely the responsibility of the authors and does not necessarily represent the official views of the National Institutes of Health. Z. Bursac and Z. Gong were supported in part by the National Institute on Minority Health and Health Disparities of the National Institutes of Health under award number NIMHD (U54MD012393), Florida International University Research Center in Minority Institutions.

[a] Department of Preventive Medicine, Department of Pharmacology, Addiction Science, and Toxicology, The University of Tennessee Health Science Center, 66 North Pauline Street, Room 649, Memphis, TN 38163-2181, USA; [b] Department of Biostatistics, Florida International University, 11200 Southwest 8th Street, Miami, FL 33199, USA; [c] Department of Preventive Medicine, University of Tennessee Health Science Center, 403 Doctor's Office Building, 66 North Pauline Street, Memphis, TN 38163, USA; [d] Department of Preventive Medicine, University of Tennessee Health Science Center, 659 Doctor's Office Building, 66 North Pauline Street, Memphis, TN 38163, USA; [e] Department of Orthopaedic Surgery and Biomedical Engineering, Joint Graduate Program in Biomedical Engineering, Campbell Clinic, University of Tennessee Health Science Center, E226 Coleman Building, 956 Court Avenue, Memphis, TN 38163, USA
* Corresponding author.
E-mail address: kderefin@uthsc.edu
Twitter: @KarenDerefinko (K.J.D.); @SarahHand (S.B.H.)

In a systematic review of studies of chronic pain patients who are prescribed opioids, rates of misuse across 13 high-quality studies ranged from 2.0% to 56.3% (95% confidence ratio [CI]: 13%–38%), suggesting that misuse of opioids may be very common.[6] Results from this study indicated that misuse took many forms across studies, including overuse, disorganized use, use for non-pain-related issues (eg, to manage anxiety), and concomitant use with alcohol or drugs. Importantly, opioid misuse is one of the criteria of opioid dependence, now described as opioid use disorder in the *Diagnostic and Statistical Manual of Mental Disorders* (Fifth Edition).[7]

Opioid misuse and opioid use disorder are likely to develop from prescribed use,[8] and evidence suggests that greater exposure is linearly related to risk of later misuse.[9,10] Exposure is measured by duration of opioid administration and strength of dose, resulting in a "cumulative exposure" per use period. Research supports the idea that increased cumulative exposure through repeated administration (refills) is associated with long-term opioid use.[9,10] For example, recent medical claims research indicates that among opioid-naïve patients (N = 536,767), those who fill opioid prescriptions 1 time are 2.9% likely to become long-term users, whereas those who fill 4 or more times are 26.1% likely to use opioids long term.[9]

Similarly, Shah and colleagues[10] examined relations between opioid prescriptions and continued opioid use in a very large sample of medical records (N = 1,294,247) derived from commercial health plan data during the years 2006 to 2015.[10] This work showed that for individuals prescribed at least 1 day of opioids, the probability of continued opioid use at 1 year was 6.0%, and those prescribed 8 days or more of opioid medication increased the likelihood of continued use at 1 year to 30%.[10] Furthermore, continued exposure to opioids can produce hyperalgesia in some patients, lowering their pain threshold, and leading them to crave more opioid analgesic.[11–14]

When considering the risk of exposure, orthopedic surgery settings are a clear point of intervention. Orthopedic surgeries are associated with the prescribing of more narcotics than any other surgical specialty,[15] particularly for total knee replacement (TKR) surgery,[16] which is associated with severe postoperative pain.[17] Research suggests that this pain tends to last for extended periods in some patients. Significant pain (visual analog scale score of >40) is reported by 44.4% of patients at 1 month after surgery, 22.6% of patients at 3 months after surgery, 18.4% of patients at 6 months after surgery, and 13.1% of patients at 12 months after surgery.[18] Management of this pain can lead to lengthy opioid exposure and repeated refills. Namba and colleagues[19] found that of 24,105 TKR patients, 9914 (41.5%) continued opioid use after 90 days.

Furthermore, the population of individuals presenting for TKR surgery is increasing at an exponential rate,[20] and research indicates a need for increased communication between surgeons and patients regarding appropriate opioid analgesic use before and after surgery,[21,22] as well as decreased prescribing practices.[4] Indeed, regulation of opioid analgesics has begun to be the norm in surgical settings. However, it is clear that regulation on the part of the surgeon is only 1 arm of protective action; it is possible for patients to present at other physician offices and request additional opioid medication in tandem with or following what is prescribed by their surgeon, thereby increasing their risk of potential opioid misuse and later opioid use disorder. An examination of outside prescribing of opioids following surgery is not yet available in the literature.

The Current Study

The authors examined controlled substance prescriptions following TKR surgery in a sample of 560 patients who received surgery at a large orthopedic clinic in the southern United States. The state's controlled substance monitoring database (CSMD) was accessed for each patient for the 12-month period following surgery to identify surgical clinic and nonsurgical clinic sources of opioid prescriptions. Descriptive data were summarized, and χ^2 analyses were conducted to evaluate significant differences in types of opioid prescribed by surgical site and nonsurgical site providers. Finally, generalized estimating equation (GEE) models were conducted for opioid prescription (yes/no) as a function of prescription source (surgical site vs nonsurgical site) adjusting for covariates, and for specific opioid prescription category as a function of prescription source (surgical site vs nonsurgical site), adjusting for covariates.

METHODS

This study was a CSMD review of prescriptions made to patients who received TKR surgery during the year 2018 at a large orthopedic clinic in the southern United States (N = 872). Of these patients, 312 received surgery in state but resided out of state, and therefore, the CSMD could not be accessed by study staff. These 312 patients were therefore excluded, resulting in a sample of N = 560. TKR patients' identifiers were obtained from medical charts and then matched with the CSMD to assess controlled substance prescription fills in the 12 months following the patients' surgery dates, and the sources of those prescriptions (surgical site or not surgical site prescriber). Patients' files were excluded if the TKR surgery did not take place during the year 2018.

Factors that could affect pain, surgical response, or prescribing were recorded in the data set as confounding variables. These factors included age, gender, race, surgical complications, comorbid pain condition, and number of knees replaced (concurrently and within the same year). Demographic data are presented in Table 1. All study procedures were approved by the university's institutional review board and the director of the orthopedic clinic.

Statistical Data Analysis

All data analyses were carried out with Rv4.0.2 and SAS/STATv14.2. Descriptive statistics consisted of means and standard deviations for continuous variables and percentages for categorical ones, respectively. In order to univariately compare conditional proportions of opioid prescriptions overall and by category between surgical sites, the authors applied the χ^2 test. Finally, they constructed 2 GEE models, 1 binary and 1 multinomial to model the odds of repeated opioid prescription over time as a function of surgical site while adjusting for other potential confounders listed above. These models accounted for clustering of prescriptions within patients and measured over time, as random effects, with independent covariance structure chosen based on best quasi-likelihood under the independence model fit metric. Associations were considered significant at the alpha level of 0.05.

RESULTS

The CSMD was the only source of prescribing data for this study; all noncontrolled substance medications prescribed were not assessed. The sample (N = 560) was primarily white (66.1%) and female (56.6%). The mean age of the sample was 65.1 years old, and the average number of prescriptions from the CSMD per patient for 12 months was 9.2. There were a total of 711 prescribers identified in the CSMD for this sample of patients. All patients presented for TKR surgery at the orthopedic clinic: 42.3% received prescriptions only from the orthopedic clinic prescriber (surgical site provider; n = 590); 3.6% received a prescription only from an outside provider (nonsurgical site provider; n = 121); and 54.1% received at least 1 prescription from both sources. Most patients received surgery on a single knee (99.1%), and very few showed surgical complications (2.0%). Table 1 presents the sample characteristics.

Of all prescriptions detected for the 12-month follow-up period on the CSMD, 64%

Table 1
Demographic characteristics of the sample

Variable	%	Mean (Standard Deviation)
Age		65.1 (10.4)
Gender, male	43.4	
Race, white	66.1	
Race, black	29.1	
Race, other	2.3	
Race, unknown	2.5	
Double knee replacement concurrent	99.1	
Complications following surgery	2.0	
Comorbid injury at the time of surgery	95.4	
Comorbid medical conditions	91.3	
More than 1 knee surgery in 12 mo (not concurrent)	12.9	
Number of controlled substance prescriptions per patient		9.2 (9.3)

were for opioid medications. When examining opioid versus nonopioid prescription rates across prescriber type, 85% of surgical site prescriber' prescriptions are opioids, versus 41% opioids for nonsurgical site prescribers (Table 2). Pearson's χ^2 test with Yates' continuity correction indicated that this difference in opioid prescribing was significant (χ^2 = 1072.8, df = 1, P<.001). Although surgical site prescribers prescribe at a significantly higher rate, patients still acquire a high proportion of opioids outside of the clinic.

When examining results by medication class, patterns for type of opioid emerged (Table 3). Compared with surgical site prescribers, nonsurgical site prescribers prescribe more hydrocodone (15% vs 7%), other opioids such as codeine (6% vs 1%), and nonopioid pain medications (59% vs 15%), whereas surgical site prescribers prescribe more oxycodone (34% vs 11%) and tramadol (42% vs 9%). These prescription rate differences across medication classes for type of provider were significant (χ^2 = 1690.7, df = 4, P<.001).

The overall GEE model confirmed that surgical site prescriber is associated with increased odds of any opioid prescription (odds ratio [OR] = 8.18; 95% CI = 6.12–10.94; P<.0001). Among other covariates, whites had 50% lower odds of obtaining an opioid prescription compared with other racial/ethnic groups (Table 4).

A multinomial model was conducted to compare 4 opioid medication classes relative to nonopioid reference group (Table 5). Results show that surgical site prescriber had much higher odds of prescribing oxycodone (OR = 12.24; 95% CI = 8.01–18.71; P<.0001) and tramadol (OR = 18.53; 95% CI = 11.68–29.40; P<.0001). Relative to nonopioids, there was also a higher likelihood of hydrocodone prescription; however, it is important to note that compared with oxycodone and tramadol, surgical site had 85% to 90% lower odds of hydrocodone and other opioid prescriptions (all P<.0001; data not shown). Surgical site was associated with 20% lower odds of other opioid

prescriptions, such as codeine, although not significant. Men had more than 2 times the odds of other opioid prescription compared with women (P = .05), In general, whites were associated with lower odds of all opioid prescriptions, especially oxycodone, hydrocodone, and tramadol (all P<.05). Complications resulted in a 2.5-fold increase in odds of other opioid prescriptions, whereas having 2 surgeries compared with 1 surgery was associated with a 60% reduction in odds of other opioids, such as codeine (both P<.05). Comorbid injury was trending toward lower odds of tramadol use, whereas other comorbidity was trending toward a 2-fold increase in hydrocodone (both P<.1). Age was not associated with any of the opioid medication classes.

DISCUSSION

The opioid crisis has alerted prescribers to the fact that close monitoring of opioid use, long-term use, and misuse is critical to thwarting later dependence, but sources of opioid prescriptions are not immediately apparent. The authors' study sought to identify the likelihood of opioid prescribing outside of the surgical setting for the 12 months following a notably painful surgery.

Results from the authors' study indicated that of all the 5164 prescriptions documented on the CSMD for these 560 TKR patients, 64% were for opioid medications. In addition, more than half of the patients received controlled substances from both the surgery site provider and a nonsurgery site provider in the year following surgery. Although surgical site prescribers prescribe at a significantly higher rate (85% vs 41%), patients still acquire a high proportion of opioids outside of the clinic.

Importantly, in cases whereby nonsurgical site prescribers prescribed opioids at higher rates, these prescriptions were for lower MME types of opioids, such as hydrocodone (MME conversion factor = 1), and codeine (MME conversion factor = 0.15), or for nonopioid medications. This finding suggests that although opioids are indeed prescribed outside of the surgical setting, nonsurgical prescribers appear to be

Table 2 Percent of controlled drug prescription that are opioids by provider		
	Controlled Substances	
	Opioid, %	Nonopioid, %
Surgical site prescribed	84.7	15.3
Nonsurgical site prescribed	40.8	59.2

χ^2 P<.0001.

Table 3
Provider type by medication class

	Nonopioid, %	Hydrocodone, %	Oxycodone, %	Tramadol, %	Other Opioid, %
Surgical site prescribed	15.3	7.3	33.7	42.5	1.1
Nonsurgical site prescribed	59.2	15.6	10.7	8.8	5.6

χ^2 $P<.0001$.

cautious in practice. However, even lower MME opioid medications can be used in higher amounts than prescribed, indicating that even this practice carries significant risk.

Generalized estimating equations developed a rich picture of other factors that accounted for opioid prescribing. Although overall surgical site prescribers prescribed more opioids, white race had *lower* odds of being prescribed an opioid in the 12 months following TKR surgery. This finding is contrary to what is usually found in the literature about racial differences in opioid receipt; it is typical for black patients to receive suboptimal pain care.[23] The multinomial model confirmed higher MME-type opioid prescribing by surgical site providers, which is intuitive given the pain experienced following TKR surgery,[16,17] and confirmed lower odds across all opioid prescription types for white patients. Interestingly, men had twice the likelihood of other opioid prescription than women. Some trends were easily understood, such as complications increasing odds for other opioid use, and comorbid medical conditions increasing odds of hydrocodone use, whereas others were difficult to contextualize, such as 2 surgeries resulting in

lower "other opioid" use, and comorbid injury reducing odds of tramadol use. It is possible in these latter cases that other medications were prescribed to manage pain, or that opioids were discontinued because of interactions with other analgesia.

For Practitioners
It is clear from these results that all providers should consider accessing the CSMD before prescribing opioid medication to ensure minimal risk of overprescribing or prescribing for long duration. Evidence of cumulative risk for developing long-term opioid use or opioid use disorder following extended exposure (through repeated refills) is abundant,[9,10] and without adequate monitoring, patients may unwittingly be increasing their risk of later issues through requests for opioid analgesic.

In addition to close monitoring of the number of opioid prescriptions that patients receive, several other practices may decrease the patient's risk. These practices include, but are not limited to, normalizing pain and managing patients' expectations of pain following surgeries, given that fear of pain and interpretation that

Table 4
Generalized estimating equation model for any opioid prescription

	Any Opioid		
	OR	95% CI	P Value
Surgical site prescriber	8.18	6.12, 10.94	<.0001
Gender (male vs female)	1.04	0.75, 1.43	.8184
Age	1.01	0.99, 1.02	.2739
Race (white vs nonwhite)	0.56	0.39, 0.79	.0012
Complications	1.51	0.75, 3.06	.253
Comorbid injury	0.81	0.41, 1.57	.5278
Other comorbidity	1.12	0.65, 1.93	.6908
Number of knee surgeries (2 vs 1)	0.77	0.46, 1.31	.3358

Table 5
Multinomial generalized estimating equation model for opioid medication class compared with nonopioid

	Oxycodone			Hydrocodone			Tramadol			Other Opioids		
	OR	95% CI	P Value	OR	95% CI	P Value	OR	95% CI	P Value	OR	95% CI	P Value
Surgical site	12.24	8.01, 18.71	<.0001	1.79	1.23, 2.59	.0023	18.53	11.68, 29.40	<.0001	0.81	0.29, 2.25	.6835
Gender (male vs female)	1.22	0.84, 1.78	.2968	0.78	0.49, 1.24	.2945	0.94	0.63, 1.39	.7463	2.18	0.98, 4.86	.0569
Age	1.01	0.99, 1.02	.4859	1.01	0.99, 1.03	.1378	1.01	0.99, 1.03	.1371	0.98	0.95, 1.01	.1918
Race (white vs nonwhite)	0.64	0.42, 0.98	.0393	0.38	0.24, 0.58	<.0001	0.68	0.46, 1.02	.0595	0.53	0.2, 1.38	.192
Complication	1.66	0.72, 3.81	.23	0.85	0.30, 2.40	.758	1.40	0.56, 3.51	.4704	2.55	1.03, 6.31	.0428
Comorbid injury	0.81	0.37, 1.78	.6002	1.94	0.56, 6.73	.296	0.63	0.37, 1.07	.0889	1.47	0.26, 8.28	.6632
Other comorbidity	1.22	0.68, 2.18	.4981	2.07	0.93, 4.62	.0761	0.88	0.48, 1.63	.6854	1.34	0.45, 4.01	.604
Number of knee surgeries (2 vs 1)	0.75	0.39, 1.39	.3597	0.84	0.49, 1.43	.527	0.87	0.41, 1.83	.7137	0.40	0.17, 0.93	.0327

pain means something is wrong can lower a patient's ability to cope. Fear may also limit patients' attempts at nonopioid pain management through rest, icing, compression, and elevation, and physical therapy exercises that follow surgery, leading to slower recovery and longer recovery periods. Thorough discussions with patients, before surgery, about pain management alternatives will enable patients to plan on alternative pain management before the experience of pain, rather than encourage these strategies in an attempt to wean them from protracted use of opioids.

Limitations and Future Directions

Although informative about trends in opioid prescriptions, this broad evaluation of prescribing necessarily sacrificed the detail available in a narrower design. For example, the authors were unable to determine why other opioids, such as codeine, were prescribed to patients in this study. Although it is possible that codeine was prescribed for reasons other than surgical pain, the results of continued opioid use following surgery are stark nonetheless, given the risks of continued, cumulative exposure. When exposed to opioids because of surgical procedures, it is advised that additional opioids are not prescribed to patients because of risk for overdose and long-term use and dependence. Future work will be required to determine whether patients receiving other opioids receive them for related or unrelated conditions. Another issue with this study is the inability to determine why some patients use less opioid following TKR. It is possible that some patients were more proactive in recovery and were willing and able to use alternative pain management techniques. Having the ability to engage in physician therapy and rest is predicated on socioeconomic status, which was also not measured here, but could be an important covariate in future studies. Opioid use is effective and not expensive, which may make it the only analgesic choice for many surgical patients.

SUMMARY

This study evaluated the occurrence of opioid prescribing within and outside of surgical site following TKR surgery using the CSMD to access controlled substances. Results indicated that although surgical site providers prescribed more opioids, the amount prescribed by nonsurgical site providers was not trivial, leading to the recommendation that providers carefully consider the possibility of outside prescribing when considering opioid analgesic for their patients.

CLINICS CARE POINTS

- Evidence of cumulative risk for developing long-term opioid use or opioid use disorder following extended exposure (through repeated refills) is abundant.
- Without adequate monitoring, patients may unwittingly be increasing their risk of later issues through requests for opioid analgesic.
- Providers should consider accessing the CSMD before prescribing opioid medication to ensure minimal risk of overprescribing.
- Thorough discussions with patients about pain management alternatives will enable patients to plan on alternative pain management before the experience of pain.

DISCLOSURE

The authors have nothing to disclose.

REFERENCES

1. Manchikanti L, Singh A. Therapeutic opioids: a ten-year perspective on the complexities and complications of the escalating use, abuse, and nonmedical use of opioids. Pain physician 2008;11(2 Suppl): S63–88.
2. Substance Abuse and Mental Health Services Administration. Results from the 2017 National Survey on Drug Use and Health: detailed tables, table 1.27a – misuse of opioids in past year and past month among persons aged 12 or older, by detailed age category: numbers in thousands, 2016 and 2017. 2018. Available at: https://www.samhsa.gov/data/sites/default/files/cbhsq-reports/NSDUHDetailedTabs2017/NSDUHDetailedTabs2017.htm#tab1-27A. Accessed September 21, 2020.
3. Cheatle MD. Prescription opioid misuse, abuse, morbidity, and mortality: balancing effective pain management and safety. Pain Med 2015;16(suppl_1):S3–8.
4. Centers for Disease Control and Prevention. CDC guideline for prescribing opioids for chronic pain. 2017. Available at: https://www.cdc.gov/drugoverdose/prescribing/guideline.html. Accessed March 13, 2019.
5. Adewumi AD, Hollingworth SA, Maravilla JC, et al. Prescribed dose of opioids and overdose: a systematic review and meta-analysis of unintentional

prescription opioid overdose. CNS drugs 2018; 32(2):101–16.

6. Vowles KE, McEntee ML, Julnes PS, et al. Rates of opioid misuse, abuse, and addiction in chronic pain: a systematic review and data synthesis. Pain 2015;156(4):569–76.

7. American Psychiatric Association. Diagnostic and Statistical Manual of Mental Disorders. 5th edition. Arlington (VA): American Psychiatric Publishing; 2013.

8. Cochran BN, Flentje A, Heck NC, et al. Factors predicting development of opioid use disorders among individuals who receive an initial opioid prescription: mathematical modeling using a database of commercially-insured individuals. Drug Alcohol Depend 2014;138:202–8.

9. Deyo RA, Hallvik SE, Hildebran C, et al. Association between initial opioid prescribing patterns and subsequent long-term use among opioid-naive patients: a statewide retrospective cohort study. J Gen Intern Med 2017;32(1):21–7.

10. Shah A, Hayes CJ, Martin BC. Characteristics of initial prescription episodes and likelihood of long-term opioid use. MMWR Morb Mortal Wkly Rep 2017;66:265–9.

11. Angst MS. Intraoperative use of remifentanil for TIVA: postoperative pain, acute tolerance, and opioid-induced hyperalgesia. J Cardiothorac Vasc Anesth 2015;29(Suppl 1):S16–22.

12. Chia YY, Liu K, Wang JJ, et al. Intraoperative high dose fentanyl induces postoperative fentanyl tolerance. Can J Anaesth 1999;46(9):872–7.

13. Guignard B, Bossard AE, Coste C, et al. Acute opioid tolerance: intraoperative remifentanil increases postoperative pain and morphine requirement. Anesthesiology 2000;93(2):409–17.

14. Collard V, Mistraletti G, Taqi A, et al. Intraoperative esmolol infusion in the absence of opioids spares postoperative fentanyl in patients undergoing ambulatory laparoscopic cholecystectomy. Anesth Analg 2007;105(5):1255–62. table of contents.

15. Volkow ND, McLellan TA, Cotto JH, et al. Characteristics of opioid prescriptions in 2009. JAMA 2011;305(13):1299–301.

16. Hernandez NM, Parry JA, Taunton MJ. Patients at risk: large opioid prescriptions after total knee arthroplasty. J Arthroplasty 2017;32(8):2395–8.

17. Allen HW, Liu SS, Ware PD, et al. Peripheral nerve blocks improve analgesia after total knee replacement surgery. Anesth Analg 1998;87(1):93–7.

18. Brander VA, Stulberg SD, Adams AD, et al. Predicting total knee replacement pain: a prospective, observational study. Clin Orthop Relat Res 2003;(416):27–36.

19. Namba RS, Inacio MCS, Pratt NL, et al. Persistent opioid use following total knee arthroplasty: a signal for close surveillance. J Arthroplasty 2018; 33(2):331–6.

20. Kurtz S, Ong K, Lau E, et al. Projections of primary and revision hip and knee arthroplasty in the United States from 2005 to 2030. J Bone Joint Surg Am 2007;89(4):780–5.

21. Chan EY, Blyth FM, Nairn L, et al. Acute postoperative pain following hospital discharge after total knee arthroplasty. Osteoarthr Cartil 2013;21(9):1257–63.

22. Bremner S, Webster F, Katz J, et al. Older adults' postoperative pain medication usage after total knee arthroplasty: a qualitative descriptive study. J Opioid Manage 2012;8(3):145–52.

23. Meghani SH, Byun E, Gallagher RM. Time to take stock: a meta-analysis and systematic review of analgesic treatment disparities for pain in the United States. Pain Med 2012;13(2):150–74.

Trauma

Trauma

Extreme Nailing or Less Invasive Plating of Lower Extremity Periarticular Fractures

Peter R. Wasky, MD, Michael J. Beltran, MD*

KEYWORDS

- Extreme nailing • MIPO • Periarticular • Distal femur • Proximal tibia • Distal tibia
- Percutaneous • Suprapatellar

KEY POINTS

- Extreme nailing requires sufficient bone to allow for multiple interlocking screws- otherwise choose a plate.
- Soft tissue injury can be more critical than the fracture pattern when determining whether to plate or nail a periarticular fracture.
- Clamps and temporary K-wires are an effective strategy to convert C type fractures into A type fractures before nailing. Then place lag or position screws to avoid crowding.

INTRODUCTION

Intramedullary nailing of periarticular lower extremity fractures is difficult, even in the hands of skilled fracture surgeons who manage these injuries on a routine basis. The further toward the articular surface the fracture extends, the more difficult the injury becomes to stabilize with a nail. These challenging fractures often benefit from stabilization with a nail when feasible, because an intramedullary nail affords load-sharing properties not seen with a load-bearing extramedullary implant, allowing for an earlier return to weightbearing, in some instances immediately after surgery.[1,2] When nailing is not possible or the load-sharing properties of a nail are unlikely to be leveraged, plating is a safe and technically simpler alternative associated with good outcomes in multiple series of patients.[3–13] The decision to use a plate or attempt an "extreme" nail for periarticular lower extremity fractures is typically multifactorial, taking into account a given fracture pattern, the quality of the soft tissue envelope, the medical condition of the patient, and the importance and necessity of earlier weightbearing; sometimes, the use of both implants is advantageous.[14]

GENERAL CONSIDERATIONS

The pattern and fracture location determines whether it is amenable to nailing. Many periarticular fractures are associated with articular fracture extension that drive surgeons to immediately assume a fracture is not "nailable" and that plating must be undertaken. However, most periarticular AO Foundation/Orthopaedic Trauma Association A type fractures and many C1 and C2 fractures can safely be managed with nailing, as long as sufficient bone is present in the articular block to allow for multiple interlocking screws and/or blocking screws to be placed for construct stability after joint reduction has occurred[3] (Fig. 1). Unlike plating, the use of a nail for an intra-articular fracture requires additional preoperative planning and different reduction and temporizing fixation techniques during surgery to ensure that implant crowding does not occur and that the lag or position screws placed to stabilize the articular surface do not block the passage of the appropriate

Department of Orthopaedic Surgery, University of Cincinnati, 231 Albert Sabin Way Room 5553, Cincinnati, OH 45267, USA
* Corresponding author.
E-mail address: mbeltran0514@gmail.com

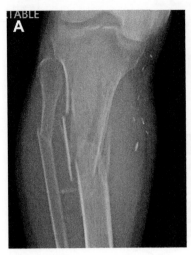
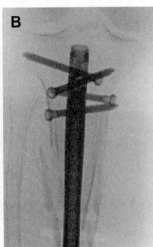

Fig. 1. (*A*, *B*) Injury radiograph and intraoperative anteroposterior (AP) view of 57-year-old patient with AO Foundation/Orthopaedic Trauma Association C2 proximal tibia fracture with extensive metaphyseal comminution. Clamping of nondisplaced articular surface allows for nail and interlocking screws to be placed. Position screws to maintain articular compression can typically be placed afterward to prevent implant crowding.

reamer trajectory, nail position, or interlocking screws.[15]

Soft tissue complications are more of a concern with plating when compared with nailing, especially of the tibia, and the condition of the soft tissue envelope must always be considered when determining an optimal treatment strategy. Even plates inserted via minimally invasive plate osteosynthesis, using small biologically friendly incisions, are associated with more soft tissue complications when compared with nails.[11,16] In evaluating the soft tissue envelope, the surgeon should take account of several important details. How swollen are the soft tissues and are blisters present? Is an external fixator in use, and if so, where are the pins located and when were they placed? Are the pin sites dry or draining? Are there traumatic open wounds present? Have fasciotomies been used to manage acute compartment syndrome and, if so, are they primarily closed or have they been skin grafted? In general, poorer soft tissues should push the surgeon to consider an extreme nail construct when able, especially in the tibia. The percutaneous incisions necessary to place nails and interlocking screws are generally not associated with significant wound complications and are not contraindicated even in the setting of severe soft tissue swelling and/or the presence of early blisters; when addressing fractures of the tibia, suprapatellar techniques allow for a portal incision to be placed more remote from the zone of injury.

Sometimes, the condition of the patient or the need for earlier weightbearing help to determine whether nailing of periarticular fractures should be performed. Older, more frail patients are perhaps the group at greatest benefit from earlier weightbearing when able.[17] Polytraumatized patients with multiple extremity fractures also benefit from earlier weightbearing. Although little high-quality, peer-reviewed literature exists to suggest improved functional outcome after immediate weightbearing of lower extremity periarticular fractures, studies of earlier weightbearing in other areas have suggested improved functional outcome measures and lower implant irritation in those patients ambulating sooner.[18] Unfortunately, there are numerous clinical situations where weightbearing will not be allowed irrespective of the periarticular fracture in question, most notably when ipsilateral fractures of the acetabulum, pelvis, or hindfoot are present.[2] In these scenarios, the decision to nail or plate should be determined based on other factors, including the fracture pattern and the condition of the soft tissues.

RELEVANT ANATOMY
Distal Femur
The morphology of the distal femur in the axial plane and the predictable deforming forces present owing to the pull of the gastrocnemius allow for reduction of many distal femur fractures using percutaneous techniques and routinely provide sufficient bone for nailing. In the axial plane the distal femur is trapezoidal, with 25° of slope medially and 10° of slope laterally; the anterior two-thirds of the condylar block is confluent with the femoral shaft and explains why precontoured distal femur plates are designed to sit more anterior on the distal femur.[5,12,19]

The gastrocnemius predictably displaces fractures in the sagittal plane by extending the condylar segment; this can be counteracted intraoperatively by using well-placed bumps, percutaneous elevators, joysticks, or a bone hook to reduce the fracture before nailing or plating. Intraoperatively, Blumensaat's line is a useful reference on the lateral view relative to the long axis of the femur, while on an anteroposterior (AP) view of the distal femur, a paradoxic notch view present should alert the surgeon to the presence of persistent recurvatum.[20]

When considering the relevant anatomy for extreme nailing around the knee, it is important to recognize that the starting point and entry reamer trajectory are paramount to ensure that the fracture remains well-reduced after nail passage. The ideal starting point for retrograde nailing is just medial to the center of the trochlea on the AP, and immediately adjacent to Blumensaat's line on a lateral view[21,22] (Fig. 2). On both views, the trajectory of the wire should be directed toward the center of the metaphysis; deviation from this trajectory is likely to induce angular deformity at the time of nail passage and may necessitate blocking screw or wire placement and rereaming to ensure an acceptable reduction.[23-26]

Proximal Tibia

The proximal tibia provides numerous insertion sites for both ligaments and tendons. Anterolaterally, Gerdy's tubercle provides for both insertion of the iliotibial band and the origin for the tibialis anterior muscle; it is a useful reference point for minimally invasive plate osteosynthesis techniques.[27,28] Because it is isometric, plates can be slid in a submuscular manner under the tibialis anterior and allowed to rest on the tubercle, often through incisions not more than 3 to 4 cm in length. The tibial tuberosity sits slightly lateral near the midline, and because of the pull of the extensor mechanism, fractures here are prone to displacement and procurvatum deformity, especially when attempting to nail.[29] The proximal tibia is wider posteriorly than anteriorly, providing large corridors of bone available for placement of oblique interlocking screws during difficult nail procedures. If nailing is undertaken, the starting point and trajectory are critically important. The ideal starting point is just medial to the lateral tibial spine on a true AP of the knee, and just anterior to the articular surface on a true lateral view[30] (Fig. 3). The trajectory should be central in the metaphysis on the AP view, and must parallel the anterior tibial cortex on the lateral view.[31]

Distal Tibia

Compared with periarticular fractures about the knee, the anatomy of the distal tibia includes much less metaphyseal bone available for purchase of screws, making nailing of very distal fracture patterns difficult. However, unlike injuries at the knee, fractures here are not predisposed to displacement owing to predictable muscular deforming forces, with malreduction usually being the result of errant guide wire placement distally and/or reaming without an

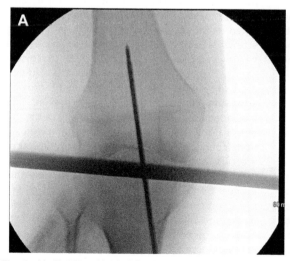
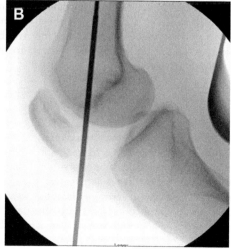

Fig. 2. (A, B) AP and lateral fluoroscopic views demonstrating appropriate starting point and trajectory for retrograde nailing. Poor starting point or irregular trajectory when nailing periarticular fractures of the knee will predispose to deformity during nail passage.

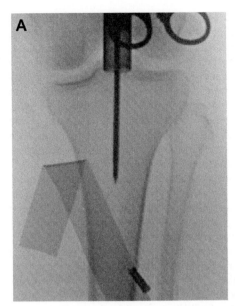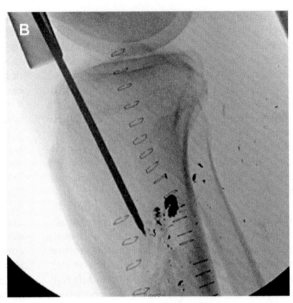

Fig. 3. (A, B) AP and lateral fluoroscopic views demonstrating appropriate starting point and trajectory for ante-grade tibial nailing. Like the femur, poor starting point or irregular trajectory will predispose to deformity during nail passage. In addition to starting point and trajectory, use of a nail with a very proximal Herzog bend will prevent posterior displacement of the distal segment, which was common with older generation nails using a more distal Herzog bend. If a suprapatellar technique is chosen, the knee must be flex 20 to 30° to obtain the appropriate wire and reamer trajectory.

acceptable reduction.[10,32–34] Avilucea and colleagues[35] demonstrated that the proximal nail insertion technique has an impact on final radiographic alignment, likely secondary to difficulty in maintaining a reduction while using the infrapatellar technique, leading to eccentric reaming of the distal segment. Finally, the physeal scar present just proximal to the articular surface must be considered when judging whether enough bone is available for nailing. Reaming through this bone is difficult in young patients and surgeons should not presume they will be able to pass the tip of the nail right up to the subchondral surface of the distal tibia.[36]

TECHNICAL CONSIDERATIONS

When a nail is chosen to manage an AO Foundation/Orthopaedic Trauma Association C type fracture, it is advantageous to open and anatomically reduce the articular surface with clamps and temporizing k-wires or lag screws, then proceed with nailing. Narrow diameter k-wires (1.6 mm, 2.0 mm) found to block the path of the reamer, nail, or lag screws can simply be moved or redirected, maintaining reduction clamps in place. After nail and interlocking screw placement, further small fragment positional screws (2.7 mm, 3.5 mm) can be placed to

maintain articular compression achieved with the clamps, safely outside of the nail and interlocking screw paths.[14]

Often more important than the presence of articular fractures, the amount of bone in the articular segment available for interlocking screw placement will usually dictate if a nail can be chosen for a given fracture. In our experience, if an articular segment allows for at least 3 points of fixation, nailing can safely be undertaken. Although having 3 or more interlocking screws is desirable, it is not always possible based on a given fracture pattern; in these scenarios, 2 interlocking screws plus the addition of 1 or more blocking screws may provide adequate construct stability and prevent late displacement.[3] In addition, the quality of the patient's bone should lend itself to optimizing fixation. Young patients with high-energy fractures are different from older patients sustaining injuries after lower energy mechanisms. The thin cortical bone seen in the metaphysis of osteopenic or osteoporotic individuals is less likely to support interlocking screw fixation, and fixation failure or late displacement is more of a concern, especially when early weightbearing is desired.[37] In these scenarios, a plate–nail combination strategy can be used to afford the early weightbearing benefits of the nail with the fixed angle stability provided by a locking plate.[14,38] Finally, it is important to recognize the implants available within a health care system. As an example, some modern retrograde femoral nails allow for up to 4 interlocking screws to be placed within 4 cm of the driving end of the nail; some or all these screws can be locked to the nail, creating a more stable fixed angle construct. These technical features allow for very extreme nailing about the knee. It is important to recognize and understand the specific implants available to you within a given medical facility, and whether implants must be brought in from outside for a given case.

The presence of an external fixator provides another challenge at the time of definitive reconstruction. Fixators in place for more than 2 weeks may predispose to deep infection when converted to an intramedullary nail, especially when the pin sites are draining.[39,40] However, this does not mean plating is always safer, because overlap of the plates with prior fixator pin sites also correlates with infection.[41,42] In general, if a fixator has been in place for less than 2 weeks, and the pin sites are well appearing, then nailing is safe to undertake. In situations where the fixator has been in place for longer than 2 weeks, especially in the tibia, a plate placed percutaneously may provide a safer alternative, and pin–plate overlap should be avoided based on pin location and fracture location, when possible. Otherwise, a pin site "holiday" may be warranted.

Proximal Tibia

Periarticular fractures of the proximal tibia have the largest body of peer-reviewed literature supporting the use of intramedullary nailing, including fractures of the proximal quarter of the bone. The technical challenges related to the nailing of these fractures, and the debate over suprapatellar versus infrapatellar nailing, have been discussed at length in both book chapters and review articles and, therefore, are not discussed at length herein. For the surgeon who recognizes the predictable deforming forces present and how to counteract them with thoughtful techniques, good reductions and patient outcomes can be expected, even with fractures involving the proximal quarter of the tibia and with articular extension.

Like the distal femur, the key determinant of whether a periarticular proximal tibia fracture can be nailed rests with determining whether sufficient interlocking fixation can be obtained in the articular block.[3] Metaphyseal comminution extending proximal to the tibial tuberosity is often

an indicator that nailing alone is unlikely to achieve sufficient fixation. Percutaneous plating is a safe alternative for these patterns, especially in the patient who will not be allowed to bear weight immediately owing to other injuries. Simple articular splits are often present (C1 and C2 fracture patterns), but usually are nondisplaced and amenable to percutaneous clamp placement and lag fixation of the articular surface away from the anticipated nail trajectory.[43,44] For extreme nailing situations with limited bone available, it is advantageous to clamp the split and not apply definitive fixation to the joint until after the nail and interlocks are placed (**Fig. 4**).

Numerous modern improvements to both tibial plate and nail systems during the past 2 decades provide for enhanced fixation options when managing very proximal fractures. Modern tibial nailing systems routinely have 4 or even 5 proximal interlocking screw options, including transverse, oblique, and anterior to posterior screw trajectories, and many holes are now threaded, allowing the screw to directly engage with the nail during insertion, improving angular stability. In addition, many systems allow for making the most proximal interlocking screw fixed angle using a "zero" locking end cap; another system allows for all 4 interlocking screws to become fixed angle when an integrated locking mechanism is engaged; this construct has been shown to be biomechanically more stable under cyclical loading compared with standard interlocking screws and still allows for later removal of interlocking screws without re-exposing the nail.[45]

Modern plating systems provide a plethora of choices when managing the proximal tibia, including monoaxial or polyaxial screw trajectories, precontoured plates for both the medial and lateral sides, and the choice between stainless steel and titanium alloy metallurgy. Implant selection becomes critical and should be tailored to a given injury. For example, if a plate and nail combination is used, polyaxial screws are likely to give the surgeon the freedom to avoid implant crowding adjacent to a nail and interlocking screws. Careful presurgical planning can also decrease interference between the screws passing through the plate and interlocking screws passing through the nail.[43] Concerns regarding galvanic corrosion of dissimilar metals may steer a surgeon toward titanium alloy plates, because all modern nailing systems use titanium alloy owing to the improved stiffness and fatigue strength profile they provide compared with older generation stainless steel nails.

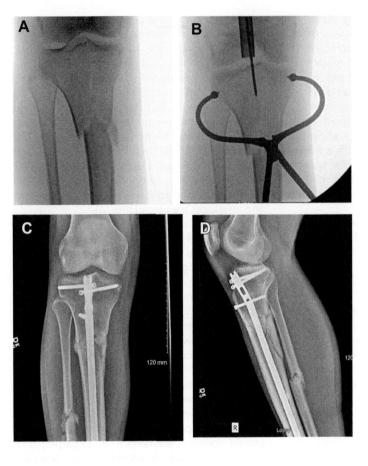

Fig. 4. (A–D) A 22-year-old male status post 30-feet fall presents with closed AO Foundation/Orthopaedic Trauma Association C1 proximal tibia fracture and ipsilateral calcaneus frac; the articular split is nondisplaced (A, B). The joint is percutaneously reduced to prevent displacement during nailing, and a blocking screw has been placed to maintain coronal alignment. The 3-month follow-up films demonstrate predictable healing of metaphysis and articular surface (C, D). In this case, independent positional screws outside the nail were not felt to be required given the patient's nonweightbearing status owing to ipsilateral hindfoot trauma.

Distal Tibia

More so than periarticular fractures of the knee, choosing to nail or plate a distal tibial fracture is highly predicated on fracture pattern and the condition of the soft tissues. Although some implants have extremely distal interlocking options—3 interlocks as close to 16 mm from the tip of the nail—in our experience it is very challenging to nail fractures that extend more than 3 cm from the articular surface, especially in young patients with a sclerotic physeal scar.

Because distal tibial fractures almost always have coronal plane malalignment, surgeons choosing to nail these injuries have the added benefit of using blocking screws to achieve stability in the coronal plane. Chan and colleagues[46] have previously shown that 2 interlocking screws plus a blocking screw was biomechanically equivalent to 3 interlocking screws under cyclical loading. Tibial nail designs typically allow for no more than 3 interlocking screws available for purchase in extreme nailing situations—2 medial-lateral holes separated by a single anterior to posterior screw option. Placing the 2 more distal

screws provides angular stability in 2 planes, with an additional blocking screw placed to prevent varus or valgus displacement based on the injury pattern. The use of 1 distal interlocking screw in the articular block is not advised because it has been shown to lead to an unacceptably high rate of nonunion.[47] When able, dual blocking screws on either side of the nail improve stability further (Fig. 5).

Because many distal tibial fractures involve metaphyseal fractures extending within a few centimeters of the articular surface, converting a C-type fracture into an A-type fracture with lag screw fixation of the articular surface first oftentimes does not make a given fracture amenable to nail fixation. In these situations, minimally invasive plate osteosynthesis techniques should be used to provide stable fixation.[32,48] Plates can safely be slid in a subcutaneous or submuscular manner through either a small medial distal leg incision or antero-laterally through a small incision using the Bohler interval; use of the latter approach requires that the plate be carefully slid up under the anterior

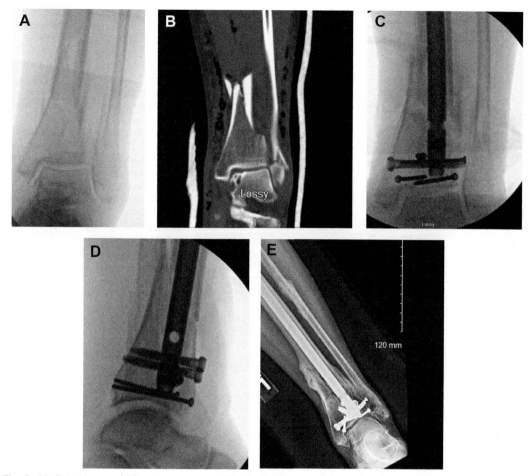

Fig. 5. (*A–E*) A 64-year-old female status post fall off a ladder, sustaining isolated open type AO Foundation/Orthopaedic Trauma Association C2 fracture of the distal tibial plafond (*A, B*). Given her soft tissue injury, she underwent a limited open reduction of the articular surface followed by extreme nailing (*C, D*). A blocking screw has been placed to augment the 2 interlocking screws to prevent late varus displacement. After nail and interlocking placement, position screws are placed to support the clamped articular surface and prevent crowding of implants. At 5 months, the fracture has progressed to union (*E*).

neurovascular bundle, which is at risk for entrapment between 4 and 11 cm above the tibial plafond.[49] With the plate provisionally fixed proximal and distal to secure length and rotation, percutaneous clamps, bumps, and other adjuvant reduction aides can be used to restore coronal and sagittal alignment before additional screws are applied above and below the fracture. Similar to techniques for true pilon fractures of the tibial plafond, percutaneous plating of metaphyseal fractures should involve placing the plate to buttress and counteract predictable planes of deformity; fractures that have failed in valgus benefit most from a laterally based plate, whereas varus modes of failure benefit from medial plates. In both instances, the soft tissues dictate what is safe and reasonable; placing an incision over highly traumatized

medial soft tissues is ill-advised and likely to lead to complications.[50,51] Associated fibular fractures, although common, do not in and of themselves warrant fixation unless associated with a rotationally unstable ankle joint (less common) or as a means of improving tibial fracture alignment and/or stability.[10,48,52,53] In 1 study, plating the fibula was associated with a higher incidence of tibial nonunion, presumably owing to decreased micromotion across the fracture leading to less predictable callous formation in cases of bridge plate fixation.[52]

DISTAL FEMUR

The distal femur remains, in our opinion, the easiest periarticular fracture to nail, even in extreme situations, including select C3-type

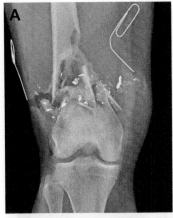
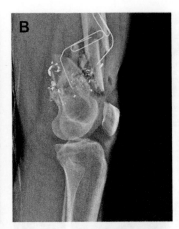
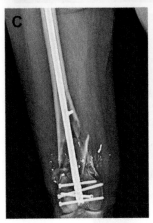
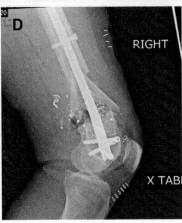

Fig. 6. (A–D) A 62-year-old female status post low velocity gunshot wound to the right thigh sustaining a highly comminuted AO Foundation/Orthopaedic Trauma Association C2 fracture (A, B). Fracture is reduced and nailed percutaneously to preserve fracture biology while restoring length, alignment, and rotation (C, D). In this case, the implant chosen allows for 4 interlocking screws to be placed within 40 mm of the driving end of the nail, allowing for sufficient distal fixation. Given the patient's age and associated medical conditions, she was permitted to mobilize immediately after surgery, and transitioned to a cane within 6 weeks of the injury.

fractures with extensive articular involvement. Because of the increased amount of bone available for screw purchase, many fractures previously only amenable to plating techniques are now safely managed with a nail in younger patients or a plate–nail combination in older more frail patients, as long as very thoughtful preoperative planning is undertaken.[14,37,38] The wide array of implant choices associated with modern nailing systems, coupled with the judicious use of blocking screws, has made it difficult to argue against nailing of distal femoral fractures unless comminution of the condyles is so extensive (most C3 fracture patterns) that interlocking screws are unlikely to achieve stable fixation.[23]

Technical planning for extreme nailing of distal femur fractures starts by determining how much bone is available for interlocking screw placement after the articular block has been reconstructed and stabilized with lag screws or, as is our preference, with provisional clamps and the judicious use of k-wires. Nailing can then be performed using percutaneous reduction techniques of the comminuted metaphysis and, after interlocking screws have been placed, positional screws can be applied to maintain the articular reductions outside of the nail and interlocking screws. If the reamer and nail trajectory must be redirected owing to angular deformity, we recommend the use of a blocking entry wire (3.2 mm terminally threaded) as opposed to a blocking screw to prevent crowding of subsequent interlocking screws. If room allows after interlocking, the wire can be exchanged for a screw to enhance stability of the construct (Fig. 6).

SUMMARY

The management of periarticular fractures of the lower extremity continues to evolve owing to improvements in surgical technique and modern implant innovation and design. The decision to attempt nailing of very proximal or distal periarticular fractures depends on several variables, including surgical skill and experience with advanced fracture techniques and concepts. Fractures not amenable to nailing are often well-suited to placement of percutaneous plates. Although early peer-reviewed evidence has emerged in support of nailing even the most complex periarticular fractures, future studies will be necessary to determine if functional and patient-reported outcomes are improved with the use of these extreme nails. Surgeons can and should continue to push the envelope regarding these injuries.

CLINICS CARE POINTS

- To avoid hardware crowding, use clamps and narrow diameter k-wires to maintain reduction of the articular block during extreme nailing, then place position screws after nail passage and interlocking to stabilize the articular surface.
- The condition of the soft tissues should always be taken into consideration when choosing a nail or a plate. Fasciotomies, compartment syndrome, prolonged use of external fixator pins, and other soft tissue injuries might favor use of a nail over a plate when possible.
- Blocking screws are effective at enhancing fixation when limited interlocking screws are available for purchase in the articular block. Place them to resist the predicted vector of displacement (review the injury radiographs)
- When nailing is not possible for a given fracture, plates are effective and can be applied via biologically friendly small incisions based on the fracture pattern.
- Nailing effectively allows for immediate or earlier weightbearing when compared with nails. If displacement is a concern with immediate weightbearing (owing to osteopenia or fracture pattern), a plate–nail combination strategy should be considered.

DISCLOSURE

Dr M.J. Beltran is a paid consultant for Smith and Nephew. Dr P.R. Wasky has nothing to disclose.

REFERENCES

1. Brumback RJ, Toal TR, Murphy-Zane MS, et al. Immediate weight-bearing after treatment of a comminuted fracture of the femoral shaft with a statically locked intramedullary nail. J Bone Joint Surg Am 1999;81(11):1538–44.

2. Kubiak EN, Beebe MJ, North K, et al. Early weight bearing after lower extremity fractures in adults. J Am Acad Orthop Surg 2013;21(12): 727–38.

3. Krettek C, Miclau T, Schandelmaier P, et al. The mechanical effect of blocking screws ("poller screws") in stabilizing tibia fractures with short proximal or distal fragments after insertion of small-diameter intramedullary nails. J Orthop Trauma 1999;13(8):550–3.

4. Ricci WM, Streubel PN, Morshed S, et al. Risk factors for failure of locked plate fixation of distal femur fractures: an analysis of 335 cases. J Orthop Trauma 2014;28(2):83–9.

5. Collinge CA, Gardner MJ, Crist BD. Pitfalls in the application of distal femur plates for fractures. J Orthop Trauma 2011;25(11):695–706.

6. Meneghini RM, Keyes BJ, Reddy KK, et al. Modern retrograde intramedullary nails versus periarticular locked plates for supracondylar femur fractures after total knee arthroplasty. J Arthroplasty 2014; 29(7):1478–81.

7. Lindvall E, Sanders R, DiPasquale T, et al. Intramedullary nailing versus percutaneous locked plating of extra-articular proximal tibial fractures: comparison of 56 cases. J Orthop Trauma 2009;23(7): 485–92.

8. Collinge C, Sanders R, DiPasquale T. Treatment of complex tibial periarticular fractures using percutaneous techniques. Clin Orthop Relat Res 2000;375: 69–77.

9. Barcak E, Collinge CA. Metaphyseal distal tibia fractures: a cohort, single-surgeon study comparing outcomes of patients treated with minimally invasive plating versus intramedullary nailing. J Orthop Trauma 2016;30(5):e169.

10. Zelle BA, Bhandari M, Espiritu M, et al. Group, on behalf of the Evidence-Based Orthopaedic Trauma Working. Treatment of distal tibia fractures without articular involvement: a systematic review of 1125 fractures. J Orthop Trauma 2006;20(1):76–9.

11. Im G, Tae S. Distal metaphyseal fractures of tibia: a prospective randomized trial of closed reduction and intramedullary nail versus open reduction and plate and screws fixation. J Trauma 2005;59(5): 1219–23.

12. Kolb K, Grützner P, Koller H, et al. The condylar plate for treatment of distal femoral fractures: a long-term follow-up study. Injury 2009;40(4):440–8.

13. Hoskins W, Sheehy R, Edwards ER, et al. Nails or plates for fracture of the distal femur? Bone Joint J 2016;98(6):846–50.

14. Liporace FA, Yoon RS. Nail plate combination technique for native and periprosthetic distal femur fractures. J Orthop Trauma 2019;33(2):e64–8.

15. Collinge CA, Beltran MJ, Dollahite HA, et al. Percutaneous clamping of spiral and oblique fractures of

the tibial shaft: a safe and effective reduction aid during intramedullary nailing. J Orthop Trauma 2015;29(6):e208.

16. Liu X, Xu W, Xue Q, et al. Intramedullary nailing versus minimally invasive plate osteosynthesis for distal tibial fractures: a systematic review and meta-analysis. Orthop Surg 2019;11(6):954–65.

17. Donohoe E, Roberts HJ, Miclau T, et al. Management of lower extremity fractures in the elderly: a focus on post-operative rehabilitation. Injury 2020; 51:S118–22.

18. Dehghan N, McKee MD, Jenkinson RJ, et al. Early weightbearing and range of motion versus non-weightbearing and immobilization after open reduction and internal fixation of unstable ankle fractures: a randomized controlled trial. J Orthop Trauma 2016;30(7):345–52.

19. Paley D. Principles of deformity correction. New York: Springer-Verlag; 2005.

20. Suk M, Desai P. Supracondylar femur fractures. In: Archdeacon MT, editor. Prevention and management of common fracture complications. Thorofare (NJ): Slack; 2012. p. 236.

21. Sanders R, Koval KJ, DiPasquale T, et al. Retrograde reamed femoral nailing. J Orthop Trauma 1993;7(4):293–302.

22. Ostrum RF, DiCicco J, Lakatos R, et al. Retrograde intramedullary nailing of femoral diaphyseal fractures. J Orthop Trauma 1998;12(7):464–8.

23. Ostrum RF, Maurer JP. Distal third femur fractures treated with retrograde femoral nailing and blocking screws. J Orthop Trauma 2009;23(9):681–4.

24. Stedtfeld H, Mittlmeier T, Landgraf P, et al. The logic and clinical applications of blocking screws. J Bone Joint Surg Am 2004;86-A(Suppl 2):17–25.

25. Rhorer AS. Percutaneous/minimally invasive techniques in treatment of femoral shaft fractures with an intramedullary nail. J Orthop Trauma 2009;23:S2.

26. Biewener A, Grass R, Holch M, et al. [Intramedullary nail placement with percutaneous Kirshner wires. illustration of method and clinical examples]. Unfallchirurg 2002;105(1):65–70.

27. Stannard JP, Wilson TC, Volgas DA, et al. Fracture stabilization of proximal tibial fractures with the proximal tibial LISS: early experience in Birmingham, Alabama (USA). Injury 2003;34:S36–42.

28. Cole PA, Zlowodzki M, Kregor PJ. Treatment of proximal tibia fractures using the less invasive stabilization system: surgical experience and early clinical results in 77 fractures. J Orthop Trauma 2004;18(8):528–35.

29. Krettek C, Gerich T, Miclau T. A minimally invasive medial approach for proximal tibial fractures. Injury 2001;32:4–13.

30. Tornetta P, Collins E. Semiextended position for intramedullary nailing of the proximal tibia. Clin Orthop Relat Res 1996;328:185–9.

31. Tornetta P, Riina J, Geller J, et al. Intraarticular anatomic risks of tibial nailing. J Orthop Trauma 1999;13(4):247–51.

32. Casstevens C, Le T, Archdeacon MT, et al. Management of extra-articular fractures of the distal tibia: intramedullary nailing versus plate fixation. J Am Acad Orthop Surg 2012;20(11):675–83.

33. Vallier HA, Le TT, Bedi A. Radiographic and clinical comparisons of distal tibia shaft fractures (4 to 11 cm proximal to the plafond): plating versus intramedullary nailing. J Orthop Trauma 2008;22(5): 307–11.

34. De Giacomo AF, Tornetta P. Alignment after intramedullary nailing of distal tibia fractures without fibula fixation. J Orthop Trauma 2016;30(10):561–7.

35. Avilucea FR, Triantafillou K, Whiting PS, et al. Suprapatellar intramedullary nail technique lowers rate of malalignment of distal tibia fractures. J Orthop Trauma 2016;30(10):557–60.

36. Schumaier AP, Avilucea FR, Southam BR, et al. Terminal position of a tibial intramedullary nail: a computed tomography (CT) based study. Eur J Trauma Emerg Surg 2020;46(5):1077–83.

37. Wähnert D, Hoffmeier KL, von Oldenburg G, et al. Internal fixation of type-C distal femoral fractures in osteoporotic bone. J Bone Joint Surg Am 2010; 92(6):1442–52.

38. Wright DJ, DeSanto DJ, McGarry MH, et al. Supplemental fixation of supracondylar distal femur fractures: a biomechanical comparison of dual-plate and plate-nail constructs. J Orthop Trauma 2020;34(8):434–40.

39. Bhandari M, Zlowodzki M, Tornetta PI, et al. Intramedullary nailing following external fixation in femoral and tibial shaft fractures. J Orthop Trauma 2005;19(2):140–4.

40. Harwood PJ, Giannoudis PV, Probst C, et al. The risk of local infective complications after damage control procedures for femoral shaft fracture. J Orthop Trauma 2006;20(3):178–86.

41. Shah CM, Babb P, McAndrew CM, et al. Definitive plates overlapping provisional external fixator pin sites: is the infection risk increased? J Orthop Trauma 2014;28(9):518–22.

42. Parkkinen M, Madanat R, Lindahl J, et al. Risk factors for deep infection following plate fixation of proximal tibial fractures. J Bone Joint Surg Am 2016;98(15):1292–7.

43. Kubiak EN, Camuso MR, Barei DP, et al. Operative treatment of ipsilateral noncontiguous unicondylar tibial plateau and shaft fractures: combining plates and nails. J Orthop Trauma 2008;22(8): 560–5.

44. Yoon RS, Bible J, Marcus MS, et al. Outcomes following combined intramedullary nail and plate fixation for complex tibia fractures: a multi-centre study. Injury 2015;46(6):1097–101.

45. Lenz M, Gueorguiev B, Richards RG, et al. Fatigue performance of angle-stable tibial nail interlocking screws. Int Orthop 2013;37(1):113–8.

46. Chan DS, Nayak AN, Blaisdell G, et al. Effect of distal interlocking screw number and position after intramedullary nailing of distal tibial fractures: a biomechanical study simulating immediate weight-bearing. J Orthop Trauma 2015;29(2): 98–104.

47. Mohammed A, Saravanan R, Zammit J, et al. Intramedullary tibial nailing in distal third tibial fractures: distal locking screws and fracture non-union. Int Orthop 2008;32(4):547–9.

48. Vallier HA, Cureton BA, Patterson BM. Randomized, prospective comparison of plate versus intramedullary nail fixation for distal tibia shaft fractures. J Orthop Trauma 2011;25(12):736–41.

49. Unlu S, Catma MF, Bilgetekin YG, et al. Minimally invasive plate osteosynthesis of distal tibia and fibular fractures through a single distal anterolateral incision. J Foot Ankle Surg 2015;54(6):1081–4.

50. Spitler CA, Hulick RM, Weldy J, et al. What are the risk factors for deep infection in OTA/AO 43C pilon fractures? J Orthop Trauma 2020;34(6):e189.

51. Gupta P, Tiwari A, Thora A, et al. Minimally invasive plate osteosynthesis (MIPO) for proximal and distal fractures of the tibia: a biological approach. Malays Orthop J 2016;10(1):29–37.

52. Collinge C, Kuper M, Larson K, et al. Minimally invasive plating of high-energy metaphyseal distal tibia fractures. J Orthop Trauma 2007;21(6):355–61.

53. Torino D, Mehta S. Fibular fixation in distal tibia fractures: reduction aid or nonunion generator? J Orthop Trauma 2016;30:S22.

Nontraditional Methods of Fibula Fixation

Casey M. Beleckas, MD, MSc[a], Jan P. Szatkowski, MD, MBA[b],*

KEYWORDS

- Fibula • Fibular fixation • Ankle fracture • Fracture fixation • Intramedullary • Rod • Nail

KEY POINTS

- Between 20 and to 30% of all ankle fractures occur in elderly patients, a population with high rates of comorbidities, impaired healing function, and low immunity.
- Traditional methods of fibular fixation are successful, but can often be plagued with complications.
- Nontraditional fibular fixation methods, such as intramedullary nail and screw fixation, are less invasive alternatives that can provide similar or improved outcomes compared with traditional methods.

INTRODUCTION

Ankle fractures represent a significant proportion of all fractures, 20% to 30% of which occur in elderly patients.[1] These fractures commonly involve the lateral malleolus, with more than 50% of ankle fractures being isolated lateral malleolar fractures in this population.[2] This rate is expected to continue to increase over the next decade.[3] In the elderly patient population, complications such as soft tissue breakdown, infection, and failure of fixation occur all too frequently.[4,5] The most traditional method of surgical stabilization of the distal fibula is plate osteosynthesis. Despite its ubiquity, different implant-related complications limit its choice as a surgical intervention in the elderly. In 1 study, 94.1% and 5.9% of the participants underwent tubular and locking plate fixation surgeries, respectively. The overall complication rate was 19.3%, among which 79.5% of the complications were minor in nature.[6] This article discusses the varied options of fibular fixation available, which may be of particular benefit in patients with poor soft tissue envelopes and/or bone quality.

Although it is clear that displaced bimalleolar and trimalleolar ankle fractures warrant operative fixation, many isolated lateral malleolus fractures may be treated nonoperatively. This is an option in most Weber A fractures, as well as some Weber B or C fractures without associated syndesmotic injury and/or deltoid incompetence.[7,8] It is crucial to assess for medial joint space widening, because there is an increased risk of fracture displacement and nonunion in the nonoperative management of unstable lateral malleolar fractures.[9] In this setting, operative stabilization of the fracture is recommended.

Traditionally, lateral malleolus fractures have been treated via open reduction and internal fixation, either with a lag screw and lateral neutralization plating or posterior antiglide plating. Lag screw fixation with neutralization plating has shown good functional outcomes for treating elderly patients with lateral malleolar fractures.[10,11] However, wound complications in an area with minimal soft tissue overlying the hardware are significant, ranging from 4.2% to 9.7%.[5,11–13] Hardware removal owing to soft tissue irritation has been reported with rates as high as 5.4%.[14] Posterior antiglide plating has also demonstrated good functional outcomes with similar wound complication rates and improved biomechanical strength.[13,15,16]

[a] Department of Orthopedics, Indiana University, 1801 N Senate Ave, MPC1 #535, Indianapolis, IN 46202, USA;
[b] Department of Orthopedics, Indiana University, IU Health, 1801 N Senate Ave, MPC1 #535, Indianapolis, IN 46202, USA
* Corresponding author.
E-mail address: jszatkowski@iuhealth.org

However, this method of fixation has also been associated with peroneal tendon irritation.[17]

In the elderly population, there is an increased concern for fracture stability in the setting of poor bone quality. Locking plates, although they have been shown to provide increased stability in the setting of osteoporotic fractures in other anatomic locations, have not demonstrated improved outcomes or increased stiffness when compared with one-third tubular plating in osteoporotic lateral malleolus fractures, while carrying similar complication rates and a higher cost.[18,19]

INTRAMEDULLARY FIXATION

Intramedullary fixation of fractures in long bones such as the femur or tibia is a common solution for fracture fixation to allow for early weight-bearing while minimizing soft tissue disturbance. Similarly, in the setting of fibular fractures, the development of intramedullary fixation has allowed for smaller incisions, frequently less than 2 cm.[20–22] This practice provides the advantage of less soft tissue stripping and, theoretically, a decreased risk of wound complications. Multiple types of intramedullary implants have been adopted for the use in fibula fractures as well as the development of novel implants for this specific indication.

RUSH RODS

Pritchett in 1993 described the use of steel rush rods in fibular fixation in unstable ankle fractures (Fig. 1). These rush rods with a diameter of 3.2 mm are inserted into the intramedullary space.[23] They are inserted from the drill hole made at the tip of the fibula. This randomized controlled trial had 25 participants, and none of them developed postoperative infections. However, all participants of this study showed nonunion, and 5 of the participants showed a poor radiologic result.

KNOWLES PIN

The Knowles pin, which has historically been used to treat intertrochanteric femur fractures, has been used for fibular fixation.[24–26] The described technique involves an open reduction, with an incision extending from 1 cm proximal to the fracture site to distal to the lateral malleolar tip.[25] An entry point 2 mm medial to the tip of the malleolus was used, followed by hand drilling and passage of a 4.0 mm threaded Knowles pin along the medullary canal path. When compared with one-third tubular plating for

lateral malleolar fractures in the elderly, similar outcomes with fewer complications (0 vs 13.3%) were found in the group treated with Knowles pins.[26]

Another study dating back to 1992 by Brown and Copus[27] shows the use of a modified Knowles pin for fibular fracture fixation. This technique involves the use of a posterolateral incision over the fracture site for reduction, which can either be extended or used as a separate incision from that created distal to the fibula to facilitate the pin's insertion. Stable reduction of the fibula must be carried out before the insertion of the intramedullary device. The modified Knowles pin is then passed through the medullary part of the distal fibula. The study done by Brown and Copus included 20 participants within the age range of 30 to 79 years. The patients presented with bimalleolar (n = 6), trimalleolar (n = 10), distal fibula (n = 4) fractures and syndesmotic injuries(n = 2). The use of modified Knowles pin in all 20 patients showed radiographic evidence of fracture union and an absence of any postoperative infection. The mean length of hospital stay after this procedure was 3.5 days with a mean time taken by the participants to achieve initial weight-bearing of 2 weeks, and full weight-bearing in 6 weeks. Three patients complained of minimal pain, and 3 complained of mild loss of plantar flexion.[27]

ELASTIC NAILS

Elastic nails have also been shown to be a viable treatment option for unstable lateral malleolus fracture (Fig. 2). The use of 2 flexible pediatric intramedullary nails to fix fibular fractures has been shown to produce favorable outcomes.[28] The use of 2 nails prevents axial rotation of the fracture when compared with screw fixation or single rod use, as well as allowing for syndesmotic fixation. The flexible nature of the nail also prevents the stress about the locking screws that is associated with rigid intramedullary fixation.[29] These are inserted from a distal entry point without reaming, most frequently with a closed or percutaneous reduction technique. Flexible nail fixation helps to avoid the incision healing complications and decreases the amount of time needed to carry out this procedure compared with traditional methods.[30] Even though the risk of malunion, nail migration, and damage to the elastic nail after trauma are considered as drawbacks of using flexible nailing, the minimally invasive nature of this process makes it a viable option

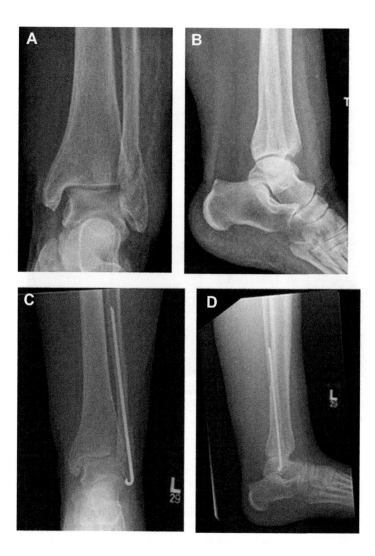

Fig. 1. Anteroposterior (*A*) and lateral (*B*) radiographs of an isolated Weber B lateral malleolus fracture in an 84-year-old woman. She was treated with closed reduction and Rush rod fixation (*C, D*).

when compared with surgical fixation with more significant risks.[21,28]

Elastic nails have also been used to treat fibula fractures in combination with fixation of tibial shaft fractures.[21,31] Wang and colleagues[21] reported good results from closed retrograde elastic nail fixation of fibular shaft fractures using 2.5- or 3.0-mm nails. No complications were reported, and good-to-excellent ankle function was reported in 95.2% of patients. Twenty percent of patients did require a small incision at the fracture site to assist with fracture reduction and/or nail passage. A case study by Simovitch and colleagues[32] in 2006 showed the benefits of using flexible titanium elastic nails in fibular fracture fixation. The use of these nails helped to preserve the length as well as treat varus and valgus displacements.[32]

A study by Yu and colleagues[31] showed the use of elastic intramedullary nails and the external fixation method (n = 27) to fix comminuted closed tibia–fibula fractures (multisegment and long spiral comminuted fractures) produces favorable outcomes in fracture fixation and faster healing of both the tibia and fibula when compared with plate fixation (n = 24) or interlocking nails (n = 29).[31] The average time taken for the participants to achieve clinical union was 11.3 ± 7.2 weeks. The fracture union rate among these 27 patients was 86.5%. In addition, 79% (22 participants) of the study population that underwent elastic intramedullary nails and external fixation achieved an excellent Johner–Wruhs outcome. This method had the lowest need for any reoperation compared with other traditional

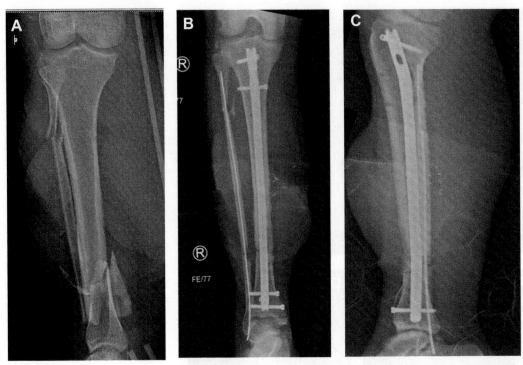

Fig. 2. A 37-year-old man presented with a segmental fibular fracture and distal third tibial shaft fracture after a motor vehicle collision (*A*). He was treated with temporary external fixation followed by delayed tibial intramedullary nailing and elastic nailing of the segmental fibula fracture (*B, C*).

methods of fracture fixation, with a complication rate of 14% (n = 4) owing to loss of reduction (n = 2), malunion (n = 1), and limb length asymmetry (n = 1).[5,31]

INTRAMEDULLARY SCREW FIXATION

Intramedullary screw fixation, similar to that used for fifth metatarsal fractures, has also demonstrated promising results (**Fig. 3**). A direct biomechanical comparison of intramedullary screw fixation versus lag screw with plate fixation has shown similar resistance to torsional loads.[33] With regard to clinical outcomes, Ray and colleagues[20] followed 24 patients treated with closed reduction and percutaneous fixation with fully threaded screws for more than 1 year. They found an average time to union of 8.2 weeks with 95.5% of the patients achieving union. The 1 incident of nonunion occurred in the setting of distraction with concomitant tibial nail placement. The average time taken by the patients to achieve full weight-bearing was 6.8 weeks. Aside from serous drainage that self-resolved, no wound complications were noted.

Other studies have also illustrated low complication rates and high union rates with the use of a screw. Smith and colleagues[34] followed 23 patients with an average age of 70 years and unstable ankle fractures with poor soft tissue and severe comorbidities. They used a 100-mm screw to fix the fibula to achieve stabilization of the unstable ankle fracture. There were no postoperative infections or signs of any nonunion. However, there were 2 complications reported, namely, screw irritation and loss of fixation. Moreover, a systemic review conducted by Loukachov and colleagues[35] on percutaneous intramedullary screw fixation in the management of distal fibula fractures found that 168 of 180 patients achieved anatomic reduction of the fracture with a low chance of complications.

Ebraheim and associates[36] conducted a study on the use of cannulated intramedullary screw fixation to manage distal fibular fractures. This study included 45 patients (mean age of 54 years) who were treated with cannulated intramedullary screw fixation method. The average time taken by the study population to achieve fracture union was 10 weeks, and the mean time to achieve full weight-bearing was

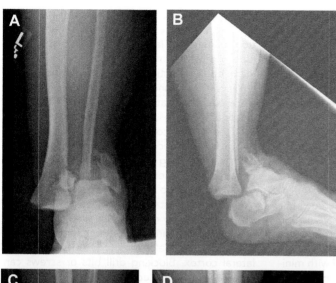

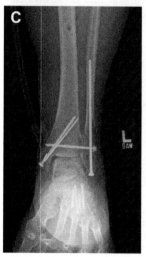

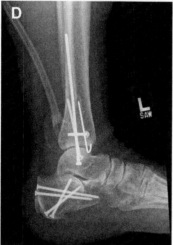

Fig. 3. Anteroposterior (*A*) and lateral (*B*) radiographs of a trimalleolar ankle fracture in a 64-year-old woman. The lateral malleolus was treated with closed reduction and intramedullary screw fixation, followed by medial malleolus fracture fixation and syndesmotic fixation (*C, D*).

14 weeks. This method showed a high union rate with few complications (4%).

FIBULAR NAILS

Over the last several years, fibula nails have become more popular, especially in the at-risk patient population. A cadaveric biomechanical comparison study by Carter and colleagues[37] in 2020 showed that intramedullary nailing is a more attractive option when compared with the locking plate fixation of unstable ankle fracture in the elderly population owing to its minimally invasive technique.

A systematic review of 17 studies on intramedullary nail fixation of fibular fractures conducted by Jain and colleagues[38] showed a mean union rate of 98% with excellent postoperative

outcome scores in 91.3% of the patients. Intramedullary fibular nail fixation also produced a significantly lower rate of postoperative complications than fixation by plating.[8] Additionally, a study conducted by White and colleagues[22] showed that there were no differences in postoperative functional outcomes, and there were fewer wound infections in ankle fractures of elderly patients treated with nail fixation.

A randomized, controlled trial with 71 patients compared the use of intramedullary nailing (Epifisa nail) versus open reduction and plating for fibular fracture fixation. Out of 71 patients, 29 participants underwent Epifisa nailing. The results demonstrated an insignificantly higher rate of bony union in nailing relative to plating (100% vs 94%). The postoperative complications were also much less frequent in nailing than plating (7% vs 45%), and function scores also favored intramedullary nailing (Kitaoka scores of 96 vs 82, where higher scores represent better function).[39] Tracey and colleagues[40] described the use of intramedullary nailing in 16 patients with distal fibula fractures with an average age of 59 years. There were no complications reported and 100% of patients achieved healing of the fracture.

In a systemic review of 8 articles on the management of patients with distal fibular fractures with minimally invasive techniques, both intramedullary nailing and intramedullary screw fixation were compared.[41] Thirty-three of 211 patients treated with intramedullary nail fixation (15.6%) exhibited complications, whereas 30 of 219 (13.7%) treated with intramedullary screw fixation and 39 of 264 (14.8%) treated with minimally invasive plate osteosynthesis had complications. The review concluded that the use of minimally invasive technique favors excellent functional results in the background of low complications in comparison with the gold standard traditional method of open reduction and internal fixation.

A randomized, controlled trial evaluating the difference between the Acumed fibular nail and open reduction and internal fixation with lag screw compression followed by neutralization plating of lateral malleolus fractures in elderly patients found a higher rate of infection in the open reduction and internal fixation group (16% vs 0%).[22] Functional scores and satisfaction were equivalent at 1 year between the groups. Despite an increase in the cost of the implant itself, the overall cost of treatment in the fibular nail group was decreased owing to fewer returns to the operating room. Errors of reduction occurred in 5 patients owing to failure to capture the distal fracture fragment or malreduction of the talus. The start point should be directly on the tip of the distal fibula aiming down the intramedullary canal. The entry reamer should be slightly medially directed to preserve the lateral cortex. Blocking drill bits or screws can be used to help redirect the guidewire and reamer as necessary.

UNSTABLE ANKLE FRACTURES WITH SYNDESMOTIC INJURY

Dabash and colleagues[24] conducted a retrospective chart review in patients (n = 18; mean age, 61 years) who underwent intramedullary

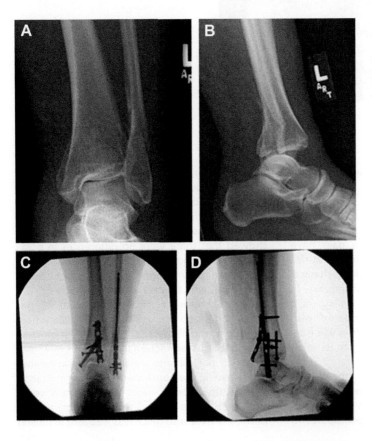

Fig. 4. Anteroposterior (A) and lateral (B) radiographs of a trimalleolar ankle fracture. The posterior malleolus was treated with open reduction and antiglide plating, followed by open reduction and locked intramedullary nail fixation of the lateral malleolus (C, D).

nail fibular fixation for unstable Weber B or C fractures. The baseline comorbidities in the patients included diabetes mellitus, advanced age, osteoporosis, and renal disease. The patients underwent syndesmotic fixation through the nail with 1 or 2 tricortical screws. Medial malleolar fixation was added for stabilization of the fractures when necessary. All patients maintained fracture reduction without failure of the syndesmotic screws. Although most patients failed to comply with the limits of weight-bearing, it neither deteriorated the prognosis of fracture reduction nor increased the risk of complications.

LOCKED NAILING

Locked nailing was developed in an attempt to combine the soft tissue preservation of intramedullary devices with a more stable fixation construct (Fig. 4). A locked fibular nail showed a greater ultimate torque to failure in biomechanical evaluation of strength than a plate and screw construct, which primarily failed owing to screw pullout.[42] In another study, biomechanical resistance to torsional loads was similar to compression screws and plate fixation.[33] Carter and colleagues[43] evaluated the risk factors for locked fibular nail device failure in a cohort of 342 patients with unstable ankle fractures. They showed that device failure rates with fibular nail fixation are only 2% and the pullout of the proximal locking screw was the primary cause of device failures. Of note, patients who developed hardware failure were on average 10 years older than the study cohort as a whole.

The Biomet locking nail has also demonstrated promising outcomes in the elderly population.[44,45] A cohort of 24 patients aged more than 70 years with lateral malleolus fragility fractures were successfully treated without any wound or hardware complications. The average time to fracture union was 8.7 weeks. This method also resulted in a higher rate of patient satisfaction and restoration of function.[45] Ramasamy and Sherry[44] reported good to excellent functional outcomes in all 11 patients in a case series of fibular nailing in Weber B ankle fractures, again with no wound healing complications.

SUMMARY

Current data suggest that ankle fractures requiring lateral malleolus fixation can result in multiple complications, especially those with poor soft tissue envelopes, open injuries, and those with compromised blood flow. Furthermore, different factors other than osteoporosis could impair the prognosis of ankle fractures in elderly patients. Patient-specific factors such as vascularity and skin lesions may prevent traditional methods of fibular fixation. As a result, nontraditional fibular fixation methods have emerged as a viable, nontraditional method for managing fibula fractures. These methods can offer comparable biomechanical strength and result in fewer potential wound complications. Early ambulation and soft tissue–friendly procedures related to fibular fixation could potentially reduce the risk of deep vein thrombosis and other problems associated with being non–weight-bearing.

The nontraditional fibular fixation methods in this review fell under the scope of intramedullary fixation and fibular nailing. The advantages provided by these methods include potential early weight-bearing, a minimization of soft tissue disturbance, and the use of smaller incisions. Several methods were described, and most studies highlighted their superiority when compared with traditional methods of fibular fixation. In various studies, the Knowles pin has shown similar outcomes with fewer complications in the elderly when compared with one-third tubular plating. Intramedullary screw fixation was found to exhibit similar resistance to torsional loads and has fewer wound complications when compared with traditional methods. Multiple studies have also pointed to the success of elastic or flexible nails in repairing fibular fractures. This method results in lower rates of infection and fewer complications overall. Patients also recover well and achieve good-to-excellent ankle function postoperatively. Locked nailing has been shown to provide superior strength over a traditional plate and screw constructs. Several studies highlight the advantages of locked nailing methods; however, 1 study did note that there were no differences in postoperative functional outcomes when comparing nail fixation to traditional methods. This finding highlights the need for further research to determine the overall effects and differences.

In conclusion, there is sufficient evidence to support the use of nontraditional methods of fibular fixation. Multiple studies from these different methods emphasize fewer complications, including wound healing, infections, and decreases in the rate of device failure. This point is particularly important in the elderly population, where many patients have comorbidities, such as diabetes mellitus, osteoporosis, and low immunity. Requiring elderly patients to undergo multiple surgeries to treat failing devices or other complications can be detrimental to their health and impact their overall quality of life. Additionally, the cost of multiple surgical procedures can be great and time consuming; thus, using nontraditional fixation methods that overall have fewer complications will be beneficial to these patients. Overall, the nontraditional fibular fixation methods discussed in this review may be suggested to improve patient prognosis and enhance the overall quality of life when treating the at-risk patient population.

CLINICS CARE POINTS

- Open treatment of lateral malleolar fractures is associated with significant wound complications.

- Intramedullary fixation such as intramedullary nails, intramedullary screws, elastic/flexible nail fixation, and rush rods allow for fibular stabilization while minimizing soft tissue disruption.

- Current evidence suggests favorable outcomes with an intramedullary nail and screw fixation of distal fibula fractures.

- Nontraditional methods that are superior to traditional plate and screw methods should be considered in specific patient populations (eg, the elderly) to improve prognosis and overall quality of life.

DISCLOSURE

The authors have nothing to disclose.

REFERENCES

1. Salai M, Dudkiewicz I, Novikov I, et al. The epidemic of ankle fractures in the elderly–is surgical treatment warranted? Arch Orthop Trauma Surg 2000;120(9):511–3.
2. Koval KJ, Lurie J, Zhou W, et al. Ankle fractures in the elderly: what you get depends on where you live and who you see. J Orthop Trauma 2005; 19(9):635–9.
3. Kannus P, Palvanen M, Niemi S, et al. Increasing number and incidence of low-trauma ankle fractures in elderly people: Finnish statistics during 1970-2000 and projections for the future. Bone 2002;31(3):430–3.
4. Zaghloul A, Haddad B, Barksfield R, et al. Early complications of surgery in operative treatment of ankle fractures in those over 60: a review of 186 cases. Injury 2014;45(4):780–3.
5. Lynde MJ, Sautter T, Hamilton GA, et al. Complications after open reduction and internal fixation of ankle fractures in the elderly. Foot Ankle Surg 2012;18(2):103–7.
6. Bäcker HC, Greisberg JK, Vosseller JT. Fibular Plate Fixation and Correlated Short-term Complications. Foot Ankle Spec 2020;13(5):378–82.
7. McConnell T, Creevy W, Tornetta P. Stress examination of supination external rotation-type fibular fractures. J Bone Joint Surg Am 2004; 86(10):2171–8.
8. Kristensen KD, Hansen T. Closed treatment of ankle fractures. Stage II supination-eversion fractures followed for 20 years. Acta Orthop Scand 1985;56(2):107–9.
9. Sanders DW, Tieszer C, Corbett B, et al. Operative versus nonoperative treatment of unstable lateral malleolar fractures: a randomized multicenter trial. J Orthop Trauma 2012;26(3):129–34.
10. Makwana NK, Bhowal B, Harper WM, et al. Conservative versus operative treatment for displaced ankle fractures in patients over 55 years of age. A prospective, randomised study. J Bone Joint Surg Br 2001;83(4):525–9.
11. Srinivasan CM, Moran CG. Internal fixation of ankle fractures in the very elderly. Injury 2001;32(7): 559–63.
12. Miller AG, Margules A, Raikin SM. Risk factors for wound complications after ankle fracture surgery. J Bone Joint Surg Am 2012;94(22):2047–52.
13. Lamontagne J, Blachut PA, Broekhuyse HM, et al. Surgical treatment of a displaced lateral malleolus fracture: the antiglide technique versus lateral plate fixation. J Orthop Trauma 2002;16(7):498–502.
14. Fenelon C, Murphy EP, Galbraith JG, et al. The burden of hardware removal in ankle fractures: how common is it, why do we do it and what is the cost? A ten-year review. Foot Ankle Surg 2019;25(4):546–9.
15. Kilian M, Csörgö P, Vajczikova S, et al. Antiglide versus lateral plate fixation for Danis-Weber type B malleolar fractures caused by supination-external rotation injury. J Clin Orthop Trauma 2017;8(4):327–31.
16. Schaffer JJ, Manoli A. The antiglide plate for distal fibular fixation. A biomechanical comparison with fixation with a lateral plate. J Bone Joint Surg Am 1987;69(4):596–604.
17. Weber M, Krause F. Peroneal tendon lesions caused by antiglide plates used for fixation of lateral malleolar fractures: the effect of plate and screw position. Foot Ankle Int 2005;26(4):281–5.
18. Davis AT, Israel H, Cannada LK, et al. A biomechanical comparison of one-third tubular plates versus periarticular plates for fixation of

osteoporotic distal fibula fractures. J Orthop Trauma 2013;27(9):e201–7.

19. Lyle SA, Malik C, Oddy MJ. Comparison of locking versus nonlocking plates for distal fibula fractures. J Foot Ankle Surg 2018;57(4):664–7.

20. Ray TD, Nimityongskul P, Anderson LD. Percutaneous intramedullary fixation of lateral malleolus fractures: technique and report of early results. J Trauma 1994;36(5):669–75.

21. Wang Q, Xu HG, Zhang YC, et al. Elastic nails for fibular fracture in adult tibiofibular fractures. Int J Clin Exp Med 2015;8(6):10086–90.

22. White TO, Bugler KE, Appleton P, et al. A prospective randomised controlled trial of the fibular nail versus standard open reduction and internal fixation for fixation of ankle fractures in elderly patients. Bone Joint J 2016;98-B(9):1248–52.

23. Pritchett JW. Rush rods versus plate osteosyntheses for unstable ankle fractures in the elderly. Orthop Rev 1993;22(6):691–6.

24. Dabash S, Eisenstein ED, Potter E, et al. Unstable ankle fracture fixation using locked fibular intramedullary nail in high-risk patients. J Foot Ankle Surg 2019;58(2):357–62.

25. Lee YS, Huang CC, Chen CN, et al. Operative treatment of displaced lateral malleolar fractures: the Knowles pin technique. J Orthop Trauma 2005; 19(3):192–7.

26. Lee YS, Huang HL, Lo TY, et al. Lateral fixation of AO type-B2 ankle fractures in the elderly: the Knowles pin versus the plate. Int Orthop 2007; 31(6):817–21.

27. Brown G, Copus A. Distal fibular stabilization with a modified Knowles pin. Iowa Orthop J 1992;12: 29–34.

28. Connors JC, Hardy MA, Ehredt DJ, et al. The use of pediatric flexible intramedullary nails for minimally invasive fibular fracture fixation. J Foot Ankle Surg 2018;57(4):844–9.

29. Megas P, Zouboulis P, Papadopoulos AX, et al. Distal tibial fractures and nonunions treated with shortened intramedullary nail. Int Orthop 2003; 27(6):348–51.

30. Crist BD, Khazzam M, Murtha YM, et al. Pilon fractures: advances in surgical management. J Am Acad Orthop Surg 2011;19(10):612–22.

31. Yu Y, Chen WK, Cui W, et al. [Minimal invasive elastic intramedullary nails and external fixation for treatment of comminuted closed fracture of tibia-fibula shaft]. Zhongguo Gu Shang 2015;28(5): 412–6.

32. Simovitch RW, Radkowski CA, Zura RD. Intramedullary fixation of fibular fractures with flexible titanium elastic nails: surgical technique and a case report. J Long Term Eff Med Implants 2006;16(2):175–8.

33. Bankston AB, Anderson LD, Nimityongskul P. Intramedullary screw fixation of lateral malleolus fractures. Foot Ankle Int 1994;15(11):599–607.

34. Smith M, Medlock G, Johnstone AJ. Percutaneous screw fixation of unstable ankle fractures in patients with poor soft tissues and significant comorbidities. Foot Ankle Surg 2017;23(1):16–20.

35. Loukachov VV, Birnie MFN, Dingemans SA, et al. Percutaneous intramedullary screw fixation of distal fibula fractures: a case series and systematic review. J Foot Ankle Surg 2017;56(5):1081–6.

36. Ebraheim NA, Vander Maten JW, Delaney JR, et al. Cannulated intramedullary screw fixation of distal fibular fractures. Foot Ankle Spec 2019;12(3):264–71.

37. Carter TH, Wallace R, Mackenzie SA, et al. The fibular intramedullary nail versus locking plate and lag screw fixation in the management of unstable elderly ankle fractures: a cadaveric biomechanical comparison. J Orthop Trauma 2020;34(11):e401–6.

38. Jain S, Haughton BA, Brew C. Intramedullary fixation of distal fibular fractures: a systematic review of clinical and functional outcomes. J Orthop Traumatol 2014;15(4):245–54.

39. Asloum Y, Bedin B, Roger T, et al. Internal fixation of the fibula in ankle fractures: a prospective, randomized and comparative study: plating versus nailing. Orthop Traumatol Surg Res 2014;100(4 Suppl):S255–9.

40. Tracey J, Vovos TJ, Arora D, et al. The Use of Modern Intramedullary Nailing in Distal Fibula Fracture Fixation. Foot Ankle Spec 2019;12(4):322–9.

41. Luong K, Huchital MJ, Saleh AM, et al. Management of distal fibular fractures with minimally invasive technique: a systematic review. J Foot Ankle Surg 2020. https://doi.org/10.1053/j.jfas.2020.05.017.

42. Smith G, Mackenzie SP, Wallace RJ, et al. Biomechanical Comparison of Intramedullary Fibular Nail Versus Plate and Screw Fixation. Foot Ankle Int 2017;38(12):1394–9.

43. Carter TH, Mackenzie SP, Bell KR, et al. Optimizing long-term outcomes and avoiding failure with the fibula intramedullary nail. J Orthop Trauma 2019; 33(4):189–95.

44. Ramasamy PR, Sherry P. The role of a fibular nail in the management of Weber type B ankle fractures in elderly patients with osteoporotic bone–a preliminary report. Injury 2001;32(6):477–85.

45. Rajeev A, Senevirathna S, Radha S, et al. Functional outcomes after fibula locking nail for fragility fractures of the ankle. J Foot Ankle Surg 2011;50(5): 547–50.

Pediatrics

Pediatric Orthopedics
Is One Fellowship Enough?

Maksim A. Shlykov, MD, MS[a], Pooya Hosseinzadeh, MD[b],*

KEYWORDS

- Pediatric orthopedic surgery • Sports medicine • Fellowship • Dual fellowship • Specialization

---

KEY POINTS

- The field of orthopedic surgery is becoming increasingly specialized, with more than 90% of residents pursuing fellowship.
- Pediatric orthopedic surgery has experienced tremendous growth in applicants and fellowship positions.
- Dual-fellowship training in pediatric orthopedics and sports medicine is emerging as a potential new subspecialty within orthopedics.
- Dual-fellowship–trained surgeons are performing an increasing percentage of total pediatric sports medicine cases.

INTRODUCTION

The breadth of the field of orthopedic surgery makes developing and maintaining in-depth knowledge and surgical skills across each discipline challenging. More than 90% of orthopedic residents currently choose to complete fellowship training in their area of interest, with some doing more than 1 fellowship.[1–3] Outside of the benefits of honing a specialized craft, fellowship training is increasingly becoming a prerequisite for jobs and an expectation from patients. Fellowship training has also been linked to improved patient-reported outcomes, decreased complications, and improved utilization of hospital-based resources.[4–6]

Although in general subspecialization within orthopedics is viewed as a positive development, it may also have negative unintended consequences. Subspecialization may leave small or underserved towns with a shortage of generalists who could be better suited to treat the vast majority of complaints within the realm of general orthopedic practice.[7] Fellowship training also may leave a growing number of surgeons feeling uncomfortable treating orthopedic problems that

are too far outside of their chosen subspecialty, which could negatively impact or delay patient care.[8] Another potential problem could be the increasing isolation of providers within their fields. Patients may need to see multiple providers over several time-consuming and potentially expensive appointments. This system also relies on effective communication between providers to coordinate patient care.[9]

Pediatric orthopedic surgery has grown rapidly over the past 2 decades, and deserves special consideration as a subspecialty. A number of articles have explored the associated changes in the pediatric orthopedic surgery workforce as it has grown; however, less has been published regarding further subspecialization within the field of pediatric orthopedic surgery.[10–13] The purpose of this article was to review dual-fellowship training and its role within pediatric orthopedic surgery.

PEDIATRIC ORTHOPEDIC FELLOWSHIP

Pediatric orthopedic surgery fellowships in North America have used the San Francisco (SF) Match Program since 2010 to coordinate

---

[a] Department of Orthopaedic Surgery, Washington University School of Medicine/Barnes-Jewish Hospital, 660 South Euclid Avenue Campus Box 8233, St Louis, MO 63110, USA; [b] Pediatric Adolescent Orthopaedic Surgery, Department of Orthopaedic Surgery, Washington University School of Medicine, 4S60, Suite 1B, One Children's Place, St Louis, MO 63110, USA
* Corresponding author.
E-mail address: hosseinzadehp@wustl.edu

Orthop Clin N Am 52 (2021) 133–136
https://doi.org/10.1016/j.ocl.2020.12.007

the fellowship match process, which has allowed for accurate tracking of fellowship data.[14] Review of SF Match data from 2011 to 2018 demonstrated that the mean number of programs and applicants has remained stable at 43 (range, 40–47) and 69 (range, 63–74), respectively. The field has grown tremendously with more than doubling of the 30 positions that were available in the late 1990s.[15] The overall match rate was 81%, with North American applicants having a match rate of 98.7% and international applicants matching at 40.9%. Unmatched positions were typically filled by applicants participating outside of the match, and between 2011 and 2014 approximately 53 to 66 spots were filled in this manner.[16] Importantly, pediatric orthopedics was found to lead the way among subspecialties, with 25% of applicants being women.[17–19]

Several studies have looked at the financial impact of fellowship training.[20–22] The most recent study by Mead and colleagues[22] found that although spine and adult reconstruction had positive net present values when compared with going straight into general practice, pediatrics and foot and ankle fellowships had negative net present values. Hand, sports medicine, and trauma fellowships were found to be neutral investments. Although the financial impact of doing multiple fellowships has not been directly studied, one could extrapolate that doing multiple fellowships may make the net present value negative for the surgeon, or make it take longer to reach a break-even point in terms of opportunity cost in lieu of general practice. The decision to pursue fellowship training should not be based on financial impact, but may be one of many factors that applicants may consider in their fellowship training choice.

MULTIPLE FELLOWSHIP TRAINING IN ORTHOPEDICS

Approximately 4% to 8% of orthopedic residents choose to perform multiple fellowships.[2,3,12] A recent study looking at American Board of Orthopaedic Surgery (ABOS) data from 2004 to 2016 found 43 different combinations of fellowships.[23] Of 9776 applicants, 444 performed multiple fellowships, with 20 applicants performing 3 fellowships and 3 applicants performing 4 fellowships. The only significant increase in fellowship combinations was for dual pediatric and sports medicine fellowships, potentially making it an emerging new subspecialty within orthopedics.

MULTIPLE FELLOWSHIP TRAINING IN PEDIATRIC ORTHOPEDICS

The trend toward additional fellowship training among applicants doing pediatric orthopedic fellowships has led to several additional studies on the topic.[10,23] Between 2005 and 2015, 45 (15%) of 310 ABOS applicants who completed a pediatric orthopedic surgery fellowship completed 48 additional fellowships; 22 (46%) of the fellowships were in sports, 8 (17%) in hand, 7 (15%) in spine, 5 (11%) in adult reconstruction, 4 (9%) in oncology, and 2 (4%) were in trauma. The investigators noted a fivefold increase in pediatric orthopedic fellowship graduates completing additional fellowships, from 5% to 28%. This is consistent with the results of a Pediatric Orthopedic Society of North America survey of recent pediatric orthopedic surgery fellowship graduates demonstrating an interest in completing at least 1 additional fellowship in 30% of graduates.[16] A separate survey identified personal interest (87%) and a competitive job market (33%) as the primary motivators for additional fellowship training.[10]

The rising popularity of dual pediatric and sports medicine fellowship training has led some to label it as a potential new subspecialty.[12] Analysis of ABOS Part II case logs from 2004 to 2014 sought to determine the volume of pediatric sports medicine cases based on fellowship completed. The percentage of cases performed by dual-fellowship–trained surgeons increased from 2.1% to 21.4% over the study period. On a per-surgeon basis, dual-fellowship–trained surgeons were found to perform 5 to 6 times as many pediatric sports medicine cases as surgeons trained in pediatrics or sports medicine alone. This is consistent with previous studies demonstrating fellowship-trained surgeons performing increasing proportions of procedures within their area of subspecialty training, with some variability between specialties.[3]

Although surgeon interest, career, and financial considerations may play a role in the decision to pursue dual-fellowship training in pediatrics and sports medicine, there appear to be patient factors that could be driving this trend. Over the past decade, operative sports injuries have increased, as has the interest of orthopedic surgeons in treating these injuries.[12] Concomitant with the increase in injuries has been an increased understanding and recognition of injuries, advancement in operative techniques for pediatric patients, and resultant comfort in treating such injuries. The potential causes of increased pediatric sports injuries are unclear, but may in part be due to increased single sports specialization at a young age.[24–27] In a survey of high school, collegiate, and professional athletes, current high school athletes who were surveyed specialized in 1 sport approximately 2 years earlier than current collegiate and professional athletes.[24] Specializing too early may put young athletes at risk for physical, emotional, and social problems. The risk of injury is typically related to overuse and affected by training volume, level of competition, and maturity.[28–35] The rise of pediatric sports medicine deserves continued monitoring through future studies.

SUMMARY

In summary, orthopedic surgery as a whole is becoming increasingly specialized. The field of pediatric orthopedic surgery has experienced significant growth over the past 20 years. Dual-fellowship–trained surgeons specializing in both pediatric and sports medicine fellowships are treating an increasing number of pediatric orthopedic injuries, making pediatric orthopedic sports medicine a potential new emerging subspecialty. With fellowship training now being the norm rather than the exception across orthopedics, it is possible that dual-fellowship training may become a prerequisite for treatment of pediatric sports medicine patients. This may impact the practices of surgeons trained in either pediatric or sports medicine alone. As the trend toward dual-fellowship training is likely to continue, future studies will be needed to characterize the impact that it has on patient care and training patterns.

DISCLOSURE

The authors have nothing to disclose.

REFERENCES

1. Daniels AH, DiGiovanni CW. Is subspecialty fellowship training emerging as a necessary component of contemporary orthopaedic surgery education? J Grad Med Educ 2014;6(2):218–21.
2. Hariri S, York SC, O'Connor MI, et al. Career plans of current orthopaedic residents with a focus on sex-based and generational differences. J Bone Joint Surg Am 2011;93(5):e16.
3. Horst PK, Choo K, Bharucha N, et al. Graduates of orthopaedic residency training are increasingly subspecialized: a review of the American Board of Orthopaedic Surgery Part II Database. J Bone Joint Surg Am 2015;97(10):869–75.
4. Althausen PL, Kauk JR, Shannon S, et al. Operating room efficiency: benefits of an orthopaedic traumatologist at a level II trauma center. J Orthop Trauma 2014;28(5):e101–6.
5. Eslam Pour A, Bradbury TL, Horst PK, et al. Trends in primary and revision hip arthroplasty among orthopedic surgeons who take the American Board of Orthopedics part II examination. J Arthroplasty 2016;31(7):1417–21.
6. Morrell NT, Mercer DM, Moneim MS. Trends in the orthopedic job market and the importance of fellowship subspecialty training. Orthopedics 2012;35(4):e555–60.
7. Sarmiento A. The projected shortage of orthopaedists may be our fault. J Bone Joint Surg Am 2012;94(14):e105.
8. Watson JT. When the iron men are all retired ... who will pin my hip? J Orthop Trauma 2009;23(2):85–9.
9. Herndon JH. The future of specialization within orthopaedics. J Bone Joint Surg Am 2004;86(11):2560–6.
10. Hosseinzadeh P, Louer C, Sawyer J, et al. Subspecialty training among graduates of pediatric orthopaedic fellowships: an 11-year analysis of the database of American Board of Orthopaedic Surgery. J Pediatr Orthop 2018;38(5):293–6.
11. Hosseinzadeh P, Obey MR, Nielsen E, et al. Orthopaedic care for children: who provides it? How has it changed over the past decade? Analysis of the database of the American Board of Orthopaedic Surgery. J Pediatr Orthop 2019;39(3):e227–31.
12. Obey MR, Lamplot J, Nielsen ED, et al. Pediatric sports medicine, a new subspeciality in orthopedics: an analysis of the surgical volume of candidates for the American Board of Orthopaedic Surgery Part II certification exam over the past decade. J Pediatr Orthop 2019;39(1):e71–6.
13. Minaie A, Shlykov MA, Hosseinzadeh P. Pediatric orthopedic workforce: a review of recent trends. Orthop Clin North Am 2019;50(3):315–25.
14. Swarup I, Luhmann S, Woiczik M, et al. Eight years of the pediatric orthopaedic fellowship match: what have we learned? J Pediatr Orthop 2020;40(2):e144–8.
15. Sawyer JR. The changing face of pediatric orthopedics. Am J Orthop (Belle Mead Nj) 2016;45(1):10–1.
16. Glotzbecker MP, Shore BJ, Fletcher ND, et al. Early career experience of pediatric orthopaedic fellows: what to expect and need for their services. J Pediatr Orthop 2016;36(4):429–32.
17. Daniels EW, French K, Murphy LA, et al. Has diversity increased in orthopaedic residency programs since 1995? Clin Orthop Relat Res 2012;470(8):2319–24.
18. Van Heest AE, Fishman F, Agel J. A 5-year update on the uneven distribution of women in orthopaedic surgery residency training programs in the

United States. J Bone Joint Surg Am 2016;98(15): e64.

19. Cannada LK. Women in orthopaedic fellowships: what is their match rate, and what specialties do they choose? Clin Orthop Relat Res 2016;474(9):1957–61.

20. Gaskill T, Cook C, Nunley J, et al. The financial impact of orthopaedic fellowship training. J Bone Joint Surg Am 2009;91(7):1814–21.

21. Inclan PM, Hyde AS, Hulme M, et al. For love, not money: the financial implications of surgical fellowship training. Am Surg 2016;82(9):794–800.

22. Mead M, Atkinson T, Srivastava A, et al. The return on investment of orthopaedic fellowship training: a ten-year update. J Am Acad Orthop Surg 2020; 28(12):e524–31.

23. DePasse JM, Daniels AH, Durand W, et al. Completion of multiple fellowships by orthopedic surgeons: analysis of the American Board of Orthopaedic Surgery Certification Database. Orthopedics 2018;41(1):e33–7.

24. Buckley PS, Bishop M, Kane P, et al. Early single-sport specialization: a survey of 3090 high school, collegiate, and professional athletes. Orthop J Sports Med 2017;5(7). 2325967117703944.

25. Feeley BT, Agel J, LaPrade RF. When is it too early for single sport specialization? Am J Sports Med 2016;44(1):234–41.

26. Myer GD, Jayanthi N, Difiori JP, et al. Sport specialization, part I: does early sports specialization increase negative outcomes and reduce the opportunity for success in young athletes? Sports Health 2015;7(5):437–42.

27. Post EG, Trigsted SM, Riekena JW, et al. The association of sport specialization and training volume with injury history in youth athletes. Am J Sports Med 2017;45(6):1405–12.

28. Brenner JS, American Academy of Pediatrics Council on Sports Medicine and Fitness. Overuse injuries, overtraining, and burnout in child and adolescent athletes. Pediatrics 2007;119(6):1242–5.

29. Brenner JS, Council On Sports Medicine and Fitness. Sports specialization and intensive training in young athletes. Pediatrics 2016;138(3).

30. DiFiori JP, Benjamin HJ, Brenner J, et al. Overuse injuries and burnout in youth sports: a position statement from the American Medical Society for Sports Medicine. Clin J Sport Med 2014;24(1):3–20.

31. DiFiori JP, Benjamin HJ, Brenner JS, et al. Overuse injuries and burnout in youth sports: a position statement from the American Medical Society for Sports Medicine. Br J Sports Med 2014;48(4):287–8.

32. Jayanthi N, Pinkham C, Dugas L, et al. Sports specialization in young athletes: evidence-based recommendations. Sports Health 2013;5(3):251–7.

33. Jayanthi NA, LaBella CR, Fischer D, et al. Sports-specialized intensive training and the risk of injury in young athletes: a clinical case-control study. Am J Sports Med 2015;43(4):794–801.

34. Luke A, Lazaro RM, Bergeron MF, et al. Sports-related injuries in youth athletes: is overscheduling a risk factor? Clin J Sport Med 2011;21(4):307–14.

35. Malina RM. Early sport specialization: roots, effectiveness, risks. Curr Sports Med Rep 2010;9(6): 364–71.

Anterior Vertebral Body Tethering for Adolescent Idiopathic Scoliosis

Early Results and Future Directions

Courtney E. Baker, MD, Todd A. Milbrandt, MD, MS,
A. Noelle Larson, MD*

KEYWORDS

- Scoliosis • Adolescent • Curve correction • Nonfusion procedure • Flexible cord • Tethering

---

KEY POINTS

- Anterior vertebral body tethering (AVBT) is a nonfusion surgical technique for correction of scoliosis in skeletally immature individuals that received US Food and Drug Administration approval in 2019 through a humanitarian device exemption.
- Curve correction occurs through 2 mechanisms: immediate intraoperative tensioning and progressive growth modulation.
- Small clinical series with midterm follow-up show AVBT corrects coronal alignment.
- Precise clinical indications, operative techniques for different scoliosis curve types, and predicted long-term outcomes are becoming clearer with more published reports.

INTRODUCTION

Scoliosis is a common condition affecting up to 1 in 300 children and can cause lifelong pain and disability. Mild curves are those less than 20°, and moderate curves are between 20° and 40°. Moderate curves between 20° and 40° in growing children can be effectively treated with bracing, which prevents curve progression but does not correct the deformity.[1] In addition, patient compliance with bracing is variable and there may be negative psychosocial consequences to wearing a brace during adolescence.

Up to 1 in 3000 children have severe scoliosis, with curves of more than 40° to 50°.[2] Severe curves more than 40° may slowly progress throughout life at a rate of 0.5° to 1° per year.[3,4] These large curves can progress throughout adulthood, resulting in deformity, pain, and potentially pulmonary complications. Abnormalities on pulmonary function testing can be detected in patients with thoracic curves

more than 70°.[5] Thus, surgical intervention is recommended for curves of more than 50° in patients who have completed their growth and for curves of more than 45° in children who are rapidly growing in anticipation that the curve will progress before skeletal maturity. In contrast with surgery in adult patients, scoliosis surgery in adolescents is thought to reduce the risk of fusion to the pelvis, is associated with less blood loss, and has fewer complications.[6]

Spinal fusion is a reliable treatment to correct scoliosis, but it has potential negative consequences. Fusion surgery involves permanently removing motion through portions of the spine, resulting in decreased spinal mobility and putting the patient at increased risk of instrumentation complications and arthritis at the levels adjacent to the fusion.[4,7] The true incidence of adjacent segment disease, degenerative arthritis, and associated disorders following childhood spinal fusion is difficult to discern.[4] Perioperative complications are common,

---

Department of Orthopedic Surgery, Mayo Clinic, 200 First Street Southwest, Rochester, MN 55905, USA
* Corresponding author. Mayo Clinic, 200 First Street Southwest, Rochester, MN 55905.
E-mail address: larson.noelle@mayo.edu

including wound infection, permanent neurologic deficit, implant problems, and blood loss requiring transfusion.[8–10]

Treatment with anterior vertebral body tethering (AVBT) is a paradigm shift for correcting Adolescent idiopathic scoliosis (AIS) using a technique similar to anterior fusion surgery to create an internal brace construct that corrects scoliosis without fusing the spine. It has been applied for roughly 10 years in an off-label manner that has precluded rigorous evaluation of the technique. In August of 2019, AVBT received US Food and Drug Administration (FDA) approval through a humanitarian device exemption, and experienced centers are now disseminating their early to midterm outcomes.[11–14] This article summarizes the basic science, early clinical reports, and future directions for this promising technique.

What Are Its Aims?

Anterior vertebral body tethering is a method of treating scoliosis through a nonfusion procedure that takes advantage of spinal flexibility and growth modulation in skeletally immature patients. The goal of AVBT is to correct scoliosis while avoiding spinal fusion, thereby maintaining spinal motion and normal articulation of the facet joints and allowing ongoing spinal growth. Compared with fusion, spinal mobility may be improved following a tethering procedure and the risk of adjacent segment arthritis in the region of the spine that is not operated on may be decreased. AVBT is an option for patients who are eligible for surgery or are at high risk of progression without the permanence of fusion. Thus, patients and families seeking an alternative to spinal fusion surgery that allows spinal growth and motion may be interested in AVBT (Figs. 1 and 2).

Current Indications

AVBT indications are broad and continue to undergo evaluation as more outcome studies with longer follow-up are published. Current FDA Humanitarian device exemption (HDE) indications are skeletally immature patients with major Cobb angles of 30° to 65° involving thoracic and/or lumbar curves for which bracing has failed or who are intolerant to brace wear. Commonly, skeletal immaturity is indicated by a Sanders bone age of 4 or less or Risser grade of 2 or less.[15] Curves of more than 65° are thought to be too severe for vertebral body tethering.

General Technique

The AVBT approach typically uses single-lung ventilation to thoracoscopically place screws into the anterior vertebral body within the thoracic space (Fig. 3). The discs are not removed and fusion is not preformed. An open approach also has been described, but there is concern that this could have deleterious effects on long-term pulmonary function. As little violation of the soft tissues around the spine as possible is made to preserve normal architecture and prevent unintended fusion. A flexible, braided polyethylene terephthalate cord is laid between the screws (Fig. 4). While the cord is placed, the patient's curve is reduced through a variety of means. Chief among them is placement of the patient in the lateral decubitus position. Additional reduction is achieved with manual tension applied through the cord after anchoring it distally, pressure placed on the convexity of the deformity, and raising the patient's legs or torso. The cord is then secured in place with standard set screws. A chest tube is maintained postoperatively to drain pleural accumulation.

Patients remain hospitalized for 2 to 4 days primarily for monitoring chest tube output as well as standard postoperative pain control, rehabilitation, and return of normal functions. Patients are expected to return to most activities at 6 weeks, and to full activities by 3 months.

Basic Science Foundation and Translational Models

In general, patients with at least 1 year of growth remaining with moderate to severe scoliosis are candidates for AVBT because curve correction occurs in 2 phases: immediate intraoperative and postoperative with growth. Immediate curve correction is achieved through the various patient positioning and intraoperative techniques. In addition, the procedure attempts to leverage the Heuter-Volkmann principle to progressively correct deformity in skeletally immature individuals (Fig. 5).[16–18] By creating compression on the convex side of the vertebra, this slows growth on the convex side and facilitates growth on the concave side of the spine.[19,20] Longitudinal growth of thoracic vertebrae has been estimated as roughly 1.6 cm/y from age 12 to 16 years.[21,22]

Since establishing the principle, physician scientists have sought to identify the most reliable technique of inducing and correcting scoliosis in various animal models (Box 1). The accumulation of this basic science solidified AVBT as a reliable means of correcting spinal deformity in skeletally immature translational models while preserving growth potential and disc health, thus creating the foundation for responsible patient trials.

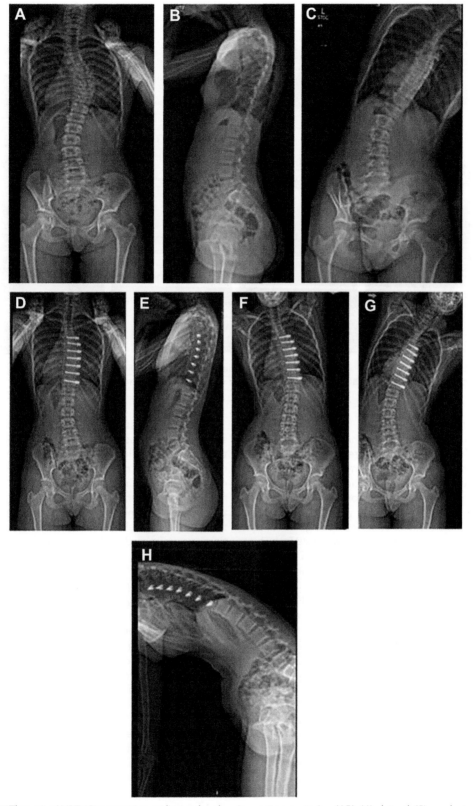

Fig. 1. Thoracic AVBT. Preoperative radiographs showing anteroposterior (AP) (*A*), lateral (*B*), and standing bending (*C*) views for evaluation of curve morphology and flexibility. Postoperative radiographs at 1 year showing AP (*D*), lateral (*E*), standing side-bending (*F*, *G*), and forward bend (*H*) views showing thoracic curve reduction and maintained spinal motion after placement of anterior lumbar vertebral body tether.

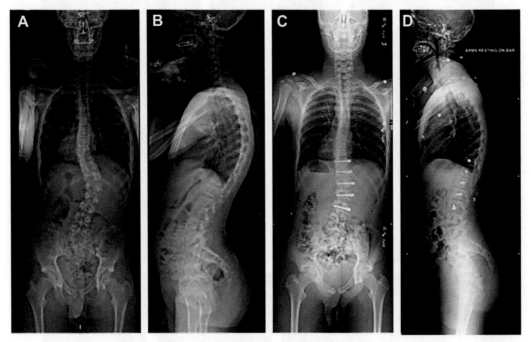

Fig. 2. Lumbar AVBT. (*A, B*) Preoperative and (*C, D*) postoperative radiographs. Full-length scoliosis views showing lumbar curve reduction after placement of anterior lumbar vertebral body tether.

Clinical Outcomes

Early human trials showed the potential efficacy and safety of AVBT for the treatment of scoliosis but were limited by small sample sizes and short follow-up timelines.[33–36] The first publication regarding human application of AVBT was a case report of a boy aged 8 years and 6 months with juvenile scoliosis in whom bracing had failed and who had had treatment with AVBT.[33] The patient's preoperative curve improved from 40° to 6° at most recent follow-up, 48 months after the index procedure, and thoracic kyphosis changed from 26° preoperatively to 18°. The patient grew 33.1 cm during this time. Although this patient was without complications 4 years after tethering, he remained skeletally immature at most recent follow-up.

Clinical series with 2 years or fewer follow-up
Samdani and colleagues[35] reported results on their first 32 patients who had AVBT with mean 2 years of follow-up. The mean age was 12 years, and the mean Sanders score was 3.2. Thoracic curve correction improved from mean preoperative magnitude of 43° to 18° at most recent follow-up. The mean compensatory lumbar curve also showed correction from 25° to 13°. One patient required bronchoscopy because of prolonged atelectasis; however, no other major complications were observed.

In 2017, Boudissa and colleagues[36] reported similar positive results in 6 patients who had tethering of the thoracic curve at a mean age of 11.2 years and mean thoracic Cobb angle of 45° and lumbar Cobb angle of 33°. At 1-year follow-up, the average thoracic curve corrected to 38° and the lumbar curve to 25°, with no patients requiring fusion. In addition, no complications were recorded in this small series of patients.

Clinical series with 2-year to 5-year follow-up
Newton and colleagues[11] presented a retrospective case series of 17 patients with 2 to 4 years of follow-up, 14 of whom had idiopathic scoliosis. Mean age at surgery was 11.2 years. The average preoperative thoracic curve was 52° and was corrected to 27° at most recent follow-up. In this cohort, revision surgery was performed in 7 patients, including 4 tether removals for complete or overcorrection, 1 addition of a lumbar tether, 1 tether replacement because of breakage, and 1 revision to a posterior spinal fusion because of curve progression. Three additional patients have been indicated for posterior spinal fusion at time of publication. Thus, a total of 10 (59%) of 17 patients either had surgery or were indicated for additional surgery.

Later, Newton and colleagues[12] retrospectively compared 23 patients with AVBT with a

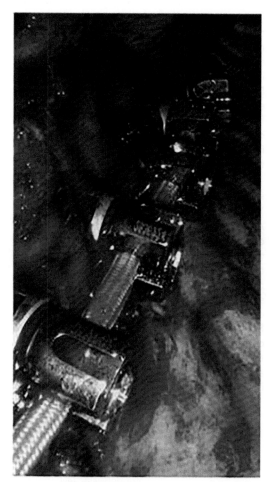

Fig. 3. In situ tether construct. Intraoperative thoracoscopic view of AVBT construct in the thoracic space.

matched cohort of 26 patients with posterior spinal fusion (PSF). Patients with AVBT were 9 to 15 years of age and Risser stage less than 2, with curve magnitudes that ranged from 40° to 67°. At mean follow-up of 3.4 years, patients with AVBT had greater residual deformity than patients with PSF (mean 33° vs 16°, P<.001). Seven patients in the AVBT cohort had 9 revision procedures, including 3 revisions to PSF, compared with no reoperations in the PSF cohort. However, patient-reported outcomes at final follow-up were similar. Curve correction and avoidance of a fusion procedure were achieved in 74% of AVBT patients in this study.

In 2020, Hoernschemeyer and colleagues[13] presented 29 patients with a mean age of 12.7 years, Sanders score of 4.3, minimum follow-up of 2 years, and mean follow-up of 3.2 years. The average main thoracic Cobb angle decreased from 50° preoperatively to 21° on first standing radiograph and 9° at latest follow-up. The investigators reported a success rate of 74%, which was defined as a residual curve of less than 30° in skeletally mature patients and no revision PSF. Two patients had PSF and 4 had tether revision, for a total 21% revision rate. In addition, 14 patients (48%) had suspected broken tethers in at least 1 location.

Also in 2020, Alanay and colleagues[14] presented similar encouraging results in 31 patients who had AVBT, specifically investigating the influence of skeletal maturity on outcomes in Lenke 1 and 2 curves. Mean age was 12 years, Sanders score was 3, and mean follow-up was 2.3 years. The average main thoracic Cobb angle was 47° preoperatively, which corrected to 22° in first erect radiographs. At final follow-up, the main thoracic curve varied by Sanders score, −3, 17, 15, 19 for Sanders 2, 3, 4 to 5, 6 to 7, respectively, and total curve correction percentage was significantly different between groups. Six patients overcorrected, 4 had pulmonary complications, and 6 had mechanical complications. Mechanical complications and overcorrection were significantly more common in the Sanders 2 cohort. The investigators recommended that AVBT be delayed, if possible, until patients are at least Sanders 3, because more skeletally immature patients showed greater risk for overcorrection and mechanical complications.

In 2019, Newton and colleagues[37] reported 4-year outcomes in a 5 patients who had AVBT with a novel device: MIScoli (DePuy Spine, Raynham, MA), which uses a braided ultrahigh-molecular-weight tether. This device technique involves no segmental compression maneuvers to gain immediate curve correction at the time of surgery. Three patients with closed triradiate cartilage (TRC) showed curve correction of nearly 15% at 4 years, whereas those with open TRC had full scoliosis correction at 2 years and overcorrection (121%) at 4 years. Greatest curve correction was noted at time of TRC closure. Two patients ultimately required revision surgery with PSF. This small series highlights that technique and timing are critical determinants of AVBT. In patients with more growth remaining (open TRC), even a tether without segmental compression can achieve complete correction and risks overcorrection.

What started as a case report in 2010 is growing into robust clinical investigation with multiple published case series in the last 3 years. The results indicate tether techniques can correct scoliosis in skeletally immature individuals and avoid fusion surgery in most treated patients. In general, case series with 2 or fewer

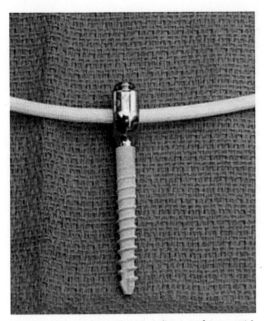

Fig. 4. AVBT implants. Screw-tether interface outside of body.

years of follow-up show encouraging coronal curve correction and minimal to no complications. Series with 2-year to 5-year follow-up show curve correction as well as complications, including reoperations and revision surgeries. Expectedly, the clinical application of AVBT is evolving as more outcome data with longer follow-up are made available. Work remains to determine the optimal treatment indications, instrumentation, and tensioning strategy for this technique.

Future Directions in Anterior Vertebral Body Tethering

AVBT is an established technique in multiple centers and stands to be widely disseminated since FDA HDE approval in 2019. Because the technique can now be studied rigorously, more retrospective series, meta-analyses, and prospective studies are certain to answer remaining questions. Four prospective surgeon-sponsored FDA investigational device exemption studies currently are underway, with plans to enroll a total of 150 patients. Further, as part of the HDE approval, the FDA states that all patients treated in the first 18-month (up to a maximum of 200

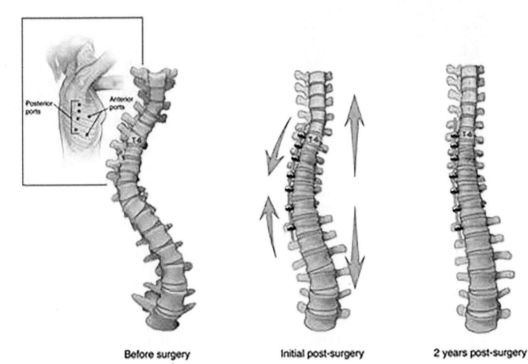

Before surgery   Initial post-surgery   2 years post-surgery

Fig. 5. Spinal application of the Heuter-Volkmann principle. Compression on the curve convexity limits longitudinal growth and enables relative lengthening of the concave side, allowing correction of spinal scoliosis. (*From* Joshi V, Cassivi SD, Milbrandt TA, Larson AN. Video-assisted thoracoscopic anterior vertebral body tethering for the correction of adolescent idiopathic scoliosis of the spine. Eur J Cardiothorac Surg 2018; 54:1134-1136. With permission from Mayo Clinic.)

Box 1
Establishment of AVBT principles

1963. Correction of spinal deformity with unilateral surgery first shown by Roaf,[23] who performed unilateral hemiepiphysiodesis in patients and achieved 10° of scoliosis correction.

2006. Braun and colleagues[24] showed tether constructs were more reliable than staples in creating spinal deformity.

2005 to 2008. In a series of translational models, Newton and colleagues[25–27] showed that asymmetric tethering was able to induce spinal curvature in a bovine model followed by a porcine model.

2008. Newton and colleagues[27,29,30] used biochemical and histologic analyses to show no change in gross morphologic disc health or disc water content after AVBT. Six months after tethering, physes on the tethered side were thinner but preserved.[27]

2013. Moal and colleagues[28] induced scoliosis by placement of a tether and then corrected the curvature by removing the tether and replacing it on the induced curve convexity.

2020. In a series of porcine experiments, Lalande and colleagues[31,32] showed predictable tension forces applied to discs and normal hysteresis disc behavior after application of tether constructs.

patients) should be enrolled and followed through 60 months from the time of each patient's index surgery, with these data reported back to the FDA initially in 6-month intervals.

The most pressing task remains solidifying surgical indications, instrumentation levels, and tensioning techniques for AVBT. Current FDA indications include AIS curves between 30° to 60°. Overcorrection remains an infrequent complication. Hoerschenmeyer and colleagues[13] showed a high success rate with more skeletally mature patients (average Sanders score 4.3), and Alanay and colleagues[14] specifically showed greater risk of complications in Sanders 2 patients. Although the translational science shows good results with guided growth, based on these preliminary reports, the clinical application seems to be more predictably successful in more skeletally mature patients.

Accurately predicting curve correction following tether procedures remains a challenge because of the many variables involved: curve magnitude, location, flexibility, skeletal maturity. Cobetto and colleagues[38] leveraged the computing power of finite element analysis (FEA) to predict patients' curve morphology 2 years after AVBT.[38] The average difference between simulation and actual Cobb angle was 4° and 5°, respectively, for immediate correction and 2-year correction. They went further to show that predicted three-dimensional (3D) correction at 2 years postoperatively varied based on cable tensioning and screw positioning.[39] For practitioners attempting to predict curve correction without the aid of FEA, Larson and colleagues[40] showed that curve magnitude in first standing erect radiographs is nearly equivalent to preoperative bending films. These data may help set postoperative expectation for both surgeons and patients.

Along with patient outcomes, best practices for intraoperative curve correction are just now being disseminated.[41,42] Multiple maneuvers can affect deformity correction intraoperatively, including patient positioning in the lateral decubitus position, bolsters and other surgical setup instruments, manual pressure on the curve apex, screw placement within the vertebral body, manual traction on the partially anchored tether, and disc release. Using FEA, Cobetto and colleagues[43] suggested that the lateral decubitus position is more effective than tether tensioning in achieving correction; they also showed that screw placement within the vertebra may differentially affect curve correction.[39] Shared outcomes of various techniques will help elucidate the safest and most effective means of obtaining curve correction.

Although animal models lend translational data supporting the safety of tethering procedures for physeal and disc health, the long-term effects of AVBT on spinal motion remain unknown. Even minor disruption of discs has been shown to induce degenerative changes,[44] and some clinicians have advocated surgical release of spinal discs for improved intraoperative surgical correction. The short-term and long-term results of such an approach are not yet available.

There also remains a disparity within the few published reports regarding success and complication rates. There is no consensus regarding the definition of success. Many investigators regard successful surgery as a residual curve of less than 35° and no conversion to PSF. Reoperation rates vary from 0% to 39%, and incidence of conversion to PSF from 0% to 13%.[12,34]

Scoliosis is a 3D deformity of the spine and, although improvements in coronal alignment have been repeatedly shown, the technique's ability to correct axial rotation has yet to be well studied. In comparison, pedicle screw fixation in PSF has impressive ability to correct scoliotic deformity in multiple planes through iterative reduction maneuvers. Future studies investigating axial deformity correction after AVBT are needed, but it is likely that patients with significant axial rotation may not experience dramatic improvement of this aspect of their scoliosis and may be less satisfied with their outcomes. At present, there are no formal indications or contraindications regarding axial rotation for AVBT patient selection. In addition, AVBT's effect on kyphosis is not fully understood. It is presumed that AVBT has a kyphogenic effect with marked kyphosis being a relative contraindication, but, theoretically, lordosis could be created with precise screw placement relative to the spine's sagittal axis. Initial reports have shown no change in the sagittal plane between preoperative imaging and latest follow-up.

Coronal overcorrection is another complication that remains incompletely understood. Several recent studies suggest that overcorrection is more likely in patients with more growth remaining.[13,14,37] From these reports, it seems that patients whose skeletal maturity is Sanders 2 or who have an open TRC are at risk for overcorrection. Correspondingly, patients with less growth remaining may be more aggressively corrected intraoperatively and do not have marked progression thereafter. Newton and colleagues[11] found that most correction occurred by the time of the first erect film, but clearly a subset of patients continue to correct well after the index surgery and even go on to overcorrect. This finding suggests that AVBT may function in 2 different ways depending on the patient's skeletal maturity: as a true growth modulator in patients with significant growth remaining or as a permanent internal brace for those nearing skeletal maturity. Clinicians may find each mechanism most appropriate for different curve types and characteristics.

In 2001, Lenke and colleagues[33,45] redefined AIS with a comprehensive classification system that aids in surgical planning and outcome research. This seminal work highlights that surgical intervention must be catered to curve pattern. Current cohorts have not studied or been powered to detect outcome differences for AVBT depending on curve type. However, Hoernschemeyer and colleagues[13] took first steps as they analyzed patients separately according to 5 subgroups. In general, they had similar improvement of both thoracic and lumbar curves across curve types. They recommended greater monitoring of patients with long thoracic curves because they may be more likely to add-on distally and require revision with PSF. Because the lumbar spine is anatomically and functionally distinct from the thoracic spine, it may become clear that surgical indications for AVBT in lumbar curves vary from thoracic curve surgical indications.

Tether breakage is a commonly reported postoperative event in AVBT series, ranging from 3% to 47%.[11,14]; however, its significance and relation to overall outcomes are not yet determined.[11,14] Neither Newton and colleagues[11] nor Hoernschemeyer and colleagues[13] regarded tether breakage as a sign of failure; however, it may be a harbinger of curves more likely to fail. Of 14 patients who had broken tethers reported by Hoernschemeyer and colleagues,[13] only half were successful, 5 were unsuccessful, and 2 had revision to PSF. In the series of Newton and colleagues,[11] 2 of 8 patients with suspected broken tethers were revised.

In addition, back pain is a common presenting complaint in adolescents with scoliosis. At this time, there is a lack of patient-reported outcomes to reliably counsel patients on how AVBT may or may not improve back pain symptoms. In their 5-patient cohort using no segmental compression technique and Ultrahigh molecular weight polyethylene tethers, Newton and colleagues[37] found that Scoliosis Research Society-22 (SRS-22) total scores decreased from 93.6 to 90.8 over 36 months; however, 2 of 5 patients were overcorrected, and this was a novel technique variant applied to a procedure still being established. Therefore, these results should not be presumed indicative of all tether procedures. More studies documenting patient-reported outcomes are critical for patient counseling.

SUMMARY

Scoliosis remains a common disorder in pediatric patients. For many years, the primary surgical treatment option has been PSF, with demonstrated long-term successful outcomes. Spinal fusion during adolescence has drawbacks of reduced growth and spinal motion and the risk of early adjacent segment disease. AVBT is a growing technique targeted for patients who are skeletally immature and desire to maintain spinal motion. It has shown early success to correct scoliosis and avoid fusion surgery, which is a major advancement in the care of AIS; however, it has shown a higher reoperation rate than PSF and long-term outcomes are yet to be defined, making appropriate patient counseling of utmost importance. The ideal surgical candidate and timing of intervention are still being determined. Patients who are motivated to maintain spinal motion can benefit from this technique. AVBT remains early in its development and best practices are beginning to be disseminated from experienced centers.

CLINICS CARE POINTS

- The AVBT approach typically uses single-lung ventilation to thoracoscopically place screws into the anterior vertebral body within the thoracic space.

- After reduction of the patient's curve through a variety of maneuvers, a flexible, braided polyethylene terephthalate cord is laid between the screw heads to maintain intraoperative curve correction.

- Case series with 2 or fewer years of follow-up report encouraging coronal curve correction and minimal to no complications; series with 2-year to 5-year follow-up have reported maintained curve correction as well as complications occasionally requiring reoperations and revision to PSF.

- Recent data suggest that AVBT outcomes may be most predictable in more skeletally mature patients, with less risk of overcorrection and mechanical complications.

DISCLOSURE

C.E. Baker has no disclosures. T.A. Milbrandt is a paid consultant to Medtronic, Orthopediatrics, and Zimmer, and holds stock in Viking Scientific. A.N. Larson has research supported by Globus Medical, Medtronic, Orthopediatrics, and Zimmer. There was no funding received for this work.

REFERENCES

1. Dolan LA, Wright JG, Weinstein SL. Effects of bracing in adolescents with idiopathic scoliosis reply. New Engl J Med 2014;370(7):681.

2. Weinstein SL. Adolescent idiopathic scoliosis: prevalence and natural history. Instr Course Lect 1989; 38:115–28.

3. Weinstein SL, Ponseti IV. Curve progression in idiopathic scoliosis. J Bone Joint Surg Am 1983;65(4): 447–55.

4. Larson AN, Baky F, Ashraf A, et al. Minimum 20-year health-related quality of life and surgical rates after the treatment of adolescent idiopathic scoliosis. Spine Deform 2019;7(3):417–27.

5. Johnston CE, Richards BS, Sucato DJ, et al. Correlation of preoperative deformity magnitude and pulmonary function tests in adolescent idiopathic scoliosis. Spine (Phila Pa 1976) 2011; 36(14):1096–102.

6. Lonner BS, Ren Y, Bess S, et al. Surgery for the adolescent idiopathic scoliosis patients after skeletal maturity: early versus late surgery. Spine Deform 2019;7(1):84–92.

7. Danielsson AJ, Nachemson AL. Radiologic findings and curve progression 22 years after treatment for adolescent idiopathic scoliosis: comparison of brace and surgical treatment with matching control group of straight individuals. Spine (Phila Pa 1976) 2001;26(5):516–25.

8. Burton DC, Carlson BB, Place HM, et al. Results of the scoliosis research society morbidity and mortality database 2009-2012: a report from the Morbidity and Mortality Committee. Spine Deform 2016;4(5):338–43.

9. Martin CT, Pugely AJ, Gao Y, et al. Causes and risk factors for 30-day unplanned readmissions after pediatric spinal deformity surgery. Spine (Phila Pa 1976) 2015;40(4):238–46.

10. Pugely AJ, Martin CT, Gao Y, et al. The incidence and risk factors for short-term morbidity and mortality in pediatric deformity spinal surgery: an analysis of the NSQIP pediatric database. Spine (Phila Pa 1976) 2014;39(15):1225–34.

11. Newton PO, Kluck DG, Saito W, et al. Anterior spinal growth tethering for skeletally immature patients with scoliosis a retrospective look two to four years postoperatively. J Bone Joint Surg Am 2018;100(19):1691–7.

12. Newton PO, Bartley CE, Bastrom TP, et al. Anterior spinal growth modulation in skeletally immature patients with idiopathic scoliosis: a comparison with posterior spinal fusion at 2 to 5 years postoperatively. J Bone Joint Surg Am 2020;102(9):769–77.

13. Hoernschemeyer DG, Boeyer ME, Robertson ME, et al. Anterior vertebral body tethering for adolescent scoliosis with growth remaining: a retrospective review of 2 to 5-year postoperative results. J Bone Joint Surg Am 2020;102(13):1169–76.

14. Alanay A, Yucekul A, Abul K, et al. Thoracoscopic vertebral body tethering for adolescent idiopathic scoliosis: follow-up curve behavior according to Sanders skeletal maturity staging. Spine (Phila Pa 1976) 2020;45(22):E1483–92.

15. Sanders JO, Khoury JG, Kishan S, et al. Predicting scoliosis progression from skeletal maturity: A simplified classification during adolescence. J Bone Joint Surg Am 2008;90a(3):540–53.

16. Mehlman CT, Araghi A, Roy DR. Hyphenated history: the Hueter-Volkmann law. Am J Orthop (Belle Mead Nj) 1997;26(11):798–800.

17. Stokes IA, Spence H, Aronsson DD, et al. Mechanical modulation of vertebral body growth. Implications for scoliosis progression. Spine (Phila Pa 1976) 1996;21(10):1162–7.

18. Akel I, Yazici M. Growth modulation in the management of growing spine deformities. J Child Orthop 2009;3(1):1–9.

19. Stokes IA. Analysis and simulation of progressive adolescent scoliosis by biomechanical growth modulation. Eur Spine J 2007;16(10):1621–8.

20. Aronsson DD, Stokes IA. Nonfusion treatment of adolescent idiopathic scoliosis by growth modulation and remodeling. J Pediatr Orthop 2011;31(1 Suppl):S99–106.

21. Dede O, Büyükdoğan K, Demirkıran HG, et al. Thoracic spine growth revisited: How accurate is the Dimeglio data? Spine (Phila Pa 1976). 2017; 42(12):917–20.

22. Dimeglio A. Growth in pediatric orthopaedics. J Pediatr Orthop 2001;21(4):549–55.

23. Roaf R. The treatment of progressive scoliosis by unilateral growth-arrest. J Bone Joint Surg Br 1963;45(4):637–51.

24. Braun JT, Akyuz E, Udall H, et al. Three-dimensional analysis of 2 fusionless scoliosis treatments: a flexible ligament tether versus a rigid-shape memory alloy staple. Spine (Phila Pa 1976 2006; 31(3):262–8.

25. Newton PO, Faro FD, Farnsworth CL, et al. Multilevel spinal growth modulation with an anterolateral flexible tether in an immature bovine model: disc health and motion preservation. Spine (Phila Pa 1976) 2005;30(23):2608–13.

26. Newton PO, Upasani VV, Farnsworth CL, et al. Spinal growth modulation with use of a tether in an immature porcine model. J Bone Joint Surg Am 2008;90a(12):2695–706.

27. Newton PO, Farnsworth CL, Faro FD, et al. Spinal growth modulation with an anterolateral flexible tether in an immature bovine model. Spine (Phila Pa 1976) 2008;33(7):724–33.

28. Moal B, Schwab F, Demakakos J, et al. The impact of a corrective tether on a scoliosis porcine model: a detailed 3D analysis with a 20 weeks follow-up. Eur Spine J 2013;22(8):1800–9.

29. Upasani VV, Farnsworth CL, Chambers RC, et al. Intervertebral disc health preservation after six months of spinal growth modulation. J Bone Joint Surg Am 2011;93a(15):1408–16.

30. Chay E, Patel A, Ungar B, et al. Impact of unilateral corrective tethering on the histology of the growth plate in an established porcine model for thoracic scoliosis. Spine (Phila Pa 1976) 2012; 37(15):E883–9.

31. Lalande V, Villemure I, Parent S, et al. Induced pressures on the epiphyseal growth plate with non segmental anterior spine tethering. Spine Deform 2020;8(4):585–9.

32. Lalande V, Villemure I, Vonthron M, et al. Cyclically controlled vertebral body tethering for scoliosis: an in vivo verification in a pig model of the pressure exerted on vertebral end plates. Spine Deform 2020;8(1):39–44.

33. Crawford CH, Lenke LG. Growth modulation by means of anterior tethering resulting in progressive correction of juvenile idiopathic scoliosis: a case report. J Bone Joint Surg Am 2010;92a(1):202–9.

34. Samdani AF, Ames RJ, Kimball JS, et al. Anterior vertebral body tethering for idiopathic scoliosis two-year results. Spine (Phila Pa 1976) 2014;39(20): 1688–93.

35. Samdani AF, Ames RJ, Kimball JS, et al. Anterior vertebral body tethering for immature adolescent idiopathic scoliosis: one-year results on the first 32 patients. Eur Spine J 2015;24(7):1533–9.

36. Boudissa M, Eid A, Bourgeois E, et al. Early outcomes of spinal growth tethering for idiopathic scoliosis with a novel device: a prospective study with 2 years of follow-up. Childs Nerv Syst 2017; 33(5):813–8.

37. Wong HK, Ruiz JNM, Newton PO, et al. Non-fusion surgical correction of thoracic idiopathic scoliosis using a novel, braided vertebral body tethering device: minimum follow-up of 4 years. JB JS Open Access 2019;4(4):e0026.

38. Cobetto N, Aubin CE, Parent S. Surgical planning and follow-up of anterior vertebral body growth modulation in pediatric idiopathic scoliosis using a patient-specific finite element model integrating growth modulation. Spine Deform 2018;6(4): 344–50.

39. Cobetto N, Parent S, Aubin CE. 3D correction over 2years with anterior vertebral body growth modulation: A finite element analysis of screw positioning, cable tensioning and postoperative functional activities. Clin Biomech (Bristol, Avon) 2018;51:26–33.

40. Buyuk AF, Milbrandt TA, Mathew SE, et al. Does preoperative and intraoperative imaging for anterior vertebral body tethering predict postoperative correction? Spine Deform 2021. https://doi.org/10. 1007/s43390-020-00267-2. Epub ahead of print. PMID: 33481215.

41. Joshi V, Cassivi SD, Milbrandt TA, et al. Video-assisted thoracoscopic anterior vertebral body tethering for the correction of adolescent idiopathic scoliosis of the spine. Eur J Cardiothorac Surg 2018;54(6): 1134–6.

42. Baker CE, Milbrandt TA, Potter DD, et al. Anterior lumbar vertebral body tethering for adolescent idiopathic scoliosis. JPOSNA 2020;2(3):1–12.

43. Cobetto N, Aubin CE, Parent S. Contribution of lateral decubitus positioning and cable tensioning on immediate correction in anterior vertebral body growth modulation. Spine Deform 2018;6(5): 507–13.

44. Nassr A, Lee JY, Bashir RS, et al. Does incorrect level needle localization during anterior cervical discectomy and fusion lead to accelerated disc degeneration? Spine (Phila Pa 1976) 2009;34(2): 189–92.

45. Lenke LG, Betz RR, Harms J, et al. Adolescent idiopathic scoliosis: a new classification to determine extent of spinal arthrodesis. J Bone Joint Surg Am 2001;83(8):1169–81.

Hand and Wrist

Hot Topics in Hand and Wrist Surgery

Travis A. Doering, MD, Benjamin M. Mauck, MD, James H. Calandruccio, MD

KEYWORDS

- Distal radius • Scaphoid • Nerve • WALANT • Flexor tendon • Basal joint

KEY POINTS

- Volar locked plating for distal radial fractures continues to demonstrate reliably good outcomes when compared with alternative techniques, including casting, but not necessarily better outcomes, and patient selection remains critical to optimizing outcomes.
- Standardized postoperative analgesia regimens simplify and minimize opioid prescriptions and may obviate altogether elective soft tissue procedures.
- The optimal treatment of scaphoid fracture nonunions remains patient and fracture specific, and although the palmar radiocarpal artery vascularized bone graft shows promising results for challenging nonunions, other data dispute the need for vascularized grafting.

DISTAL RADIAL FRACTURES

The optimal management of distal radial fractures continues to evolve. A recent meta-analysis of several high-quality randomized trials comparing operative management with volar locked plating (VLP) to nonoperative management with closed reduction and casting in elderly patients (>60 years of age) found a small but significant improvement in Disabilities of the Arm, Shoulder, and Hand (DASH) scores for the VLP group.[1] However, this DASH score difference (5.9 points) only approaches the minimal clinically important difference (7.9), so this difference should be carefully interpreted.[2] There was a larger magnitude of difference in favor of the VLP group at 3 months, and improved volar tilt, radial inclination, and supination, but these improved indices may not translate to improved function, and so a careful assessment of a patient's physiologic age, comorbidities, and social situation remains crucial to surgical indication for elderly patients with displaced distal radius fractures. However, although most patients recover well, Landgren and colleagues evaluated a subgroup of patients treated either operatively or nonoperatively that had poor outcomes at 1 year following injury.[3] Within this group (27% of 269 were treated operatively), more than half continued to have "major disability" throughout the subsequent 2- to 12-year follow-up, suggesting that regardless of treatment, disability at 1 year is likely to persist. Thus, for patients with poor outcomes following nonoperative management, earlier transition to surgical correction may prove beneficial. Identification of which patients are likely to benefit from surgery remains challenging, but Symonette and colleagues noted that for patients older than 65 years, dorsal tilt of greater than 15°, or radial inclination of less than 20°, patient-reported wrist and elbow scores were predictive of worse outcomes at 1 year. In addition, the WRIST (Wrist and Radius Injury Surgical Trial) group continues to add to the knowledge: based on 1-year postinjury Michigan Hand Outcomes Questionnaire scores, predictors of worse outcome were younger age, lower levels of education, worse pain following reduction, and more medical comorbidities.[4]

Once the decision on how to manage a distal radius fracture has been made, several recent publications can guide treatment. A prospective randomized trial of patients older than 55 years

Department of Orthopaedic Surgery and Biomedical Engineering, University of Tennessee–Campbell Clinic, 1211 Union Avenue, Suite 500, Memphis, TN 38104, USA
E-mail address: tdoering@campbellclinic.com

Orthop Clin N Am 52 (2021) 149–155
https://doi.org/10.1016/j.ocl.2021.01.004
0030-5898/21/© 2021 Elsevier Inc. All rights reserved.

of age showed that, although nonoperative management following appropriate closed reduction with a long arm plaster cast improved radiographic volar tilt, use of a short arm cast was better tolerated without other radiographic or clinical differences, leading the investigators to conclude that use of a short arm cast is appropriate.[5] Although VLP has become the standard of care, several well-performed randomized studies have examined VLP versus alternative surgical techniques, including fragment-specific plating,[6] radial column plating,[7] external fixation,[8] and percutaneous pinning.[9] Each technique has its own merits and may be favored over VLP in specific circumstances with the expectation of good outcomes in appropriately selected patients. Following surgery, although about 80% of patients participate in physical therapy, patient-reported outcomes are the same for patients who do or do not undergo formal physical therapy.[10] However, patients who undergo no formal physical therapy have greater grip strength than those who do, and patients who attend physical therapy for shorter durations reported greater function, ability to work, and satisfaction, suggesting that there may be a selection bias.

ANALGESIA IN HAND SURGERY

In 2018, 10.3 million Americans misused prescription opioids.[11] A growing appreciation of the opioid crisis has led to increased scrutiny of perioperative analgesia and pain management. Although a change in behavior might be difficult, especially given survey results suggesting that 28% of patients believe opioids are necessary for pain control,[12] it is imperative for hand surgeons to be judicious in their use and aware of alternatives. A standardized prescribing protocol has been shown to reliably reduce the number of morphine equivalents prescribed following hand surgery by 53%,[13] and alternative postoperative analgesia regimens with nonopioid medications (such as acetaminophen or nonsteroidal anti-inflammatory drugs) have been shown to afford similar levels of pain reduction after soft tissue procedures.[14] Another trial evaluating opioid reduction techniques following open carpal tunnel release (CTR) or VLP for distal radius fractures found that their reduction strategies reduced prescribed pills to 10 from 22 following CTR (with an average of 3 pills actually consumed), and to 25 from 39 pills prescribed following VLP (with 16 actually pills consumed).[15]

An alternative method to minimize opioid consumption during the opioid epidemic is the use of wide-awake local anesthesia no tourniquet (WALANT) hand surgery. WALANT has many purported advantages over other forms of anesthesia, including faster recovery, lower cost, and improved patient safety. A survey of the American Society for Surgery of the Hand members indicates that 79% had performed at least 1 WALANT procedure, and 62% actively incorporate it into their practice.[16] A prospective evaluation of WALANT versus monitored anesthesia care CTR identified that 5.5 less mean morphine equivalents (MME) were prescribed following WALANT, and that 3.6 more MMEs remained at patient's first postoperative visit.[17]

BASAL JOINT ARTHRITIS

Since the first description of trapeziectomy by Gervis in 1949,[18] a wide range of surgical solutions for arthritis of the thumb carpometacarpal joint has been proposed, and the continued variety of techniques suggests this remains an unsolved problem. Overall, regardless of technique, reconstructive surgery for arthritis at the base of the thumb is generally successful. In a single-center retrospective review with at least 1 year of follow-up, 686 operations were performed by several surgeons using a variety of techniques, and only 10 (1.5%) required early unplanned reoperation, of which only 4 required a revision arthroplasty because of pain from subsidence.[19] A systematic review of long-term outcomes following basal joint surgery suggests that failure rates are significantly higher for implant-based arthroplasties than those not requiring implants: the implant arthroplasty failure rates per 100 procedure-years were total joint replacement (2.4), hemiarthroplasty (2.5), interposition with partial trapezial resection (4.5), interposition with complete trapezial resection (1.7), and interposition with no trapezial resection (4.5). The nonimplant arthroplasty failure rates per 100 procedure-years were as follows: trapeziectomy (0.49), joint fusion (0.52), and trapeziectomy with ligament reconstruction with/without tendon interposition (0.23).[20] On account of the improved long-term durability for nonimplant procedures, and because of implant cost concerns, a "suspensionplasty" procedure was described in which a suture-based sling is created between the Flexor Carpi Radialis (FCR) and Abductor Pollicis Longus (APL) tendons to limit subsidence following trapeziectomy.[21] The APL-FCR suture suspensionplasty has been evaluated by several investigators, the largest study of which was by Weiss and colleagues, who performed this procedure in 320 thumbs and showed that it was safe (2 revision arthroplasties for subsidence), effective (complete pain relief in 84%), and functional (all working patients were able to return to their jobs).[22] Use of suture buttons and suture anchors may help the radiographic appearance following surgery, but techniques incorporating these implants have yet to demonstrate a true clinical advantage.

SCAPHOID

Although it is challenging to extrapolate economic impact from one country's health system to another's, the SMaRT trial in the United Kingdom prospectively and randomly evaluated use of immediate MRI in the emergency department to detect suspected radiographic-negative scaphoid fractures and found significant cost savings, improved detection of both scaphoid and other wrist fractures, and improved patient satisfaction.[23] Ideal management of acute nondisplaced scaphoid waist fractures remains unclear: although conservative management leads to reliable union, as the SWIFFT trial demonstrates, with a nonunion rate of 4.1% in the cast group and a number needed to treat of 44 for the percutaneous screw fixation group (44 patients with a nondisplaced scaphoid waist fracture treated to prevent 1 nonunion over casting alone at 52 weeks),[24] the earlier return to work and athletic activities enabled following screw fixation makes this attractive for select demographics.[25] However, given the higher complication rate and rate of degenerative changes at the sternoclavicular joint following operative fixation, most patients would be well treated by a short arm cast with the thumb excluded, as randomized trials have shown a standard below elbow cast without thumb immobilization sufficient for reliable healing.[26]

In fact, short arm casting has the potential to treat subacute scaphoid fractures as well: Grewal and colleagues retrospectively reviewed a series of initially untreated fractures that presented at an average of 10.5 weeks, who were then treated with casting alone. Computed tomographic evaluation identified a union rate of 82%, which increased to 96% when patients with diabetes, comminution, or a humpback deformity present were excluded.[27] However, many surgeons would treat such fractures with screw fixation, and careful methodological examination of how scaphoid union is defined remains vital when comparing results from different studies. Recent biomechanics

studies have demonstrated superior stability, stiffness, and energy absorption of both locked plating or a 2 headless-screw construct over a single-screw construction in a scaphoid nonunion model[28]; however, given the high union rate of a single-screw construct in fractures without AVN, instability, or a humpback deformity, this second screw may limit surface area for bony healing. For scaphoid nonunions, the ideal treatment is highly dependent on the individual patient and their fracture morphology. Alternative fixation constructs, including volar locked plating, as well as both local pedicled and free vascularized bone grafting may be necessary. However, the need for vascularized bone grafting at all is still in question given the results of Rancy and colleagues, who successfully treated a series of 35 proximal pole nonunions with nonvascularized bone grafting and headless compression screw fixation despite evidence of 28/33 lacking punctate bleeding and 9/23 having AVN on MRI, with 33/35 uniting by 3 months.[29] However, for the most challenging subgroup of patients with an unstable fracture, the presence of a humpback deformity and proximal pole AVN, the pedicled palmar radiocarpal artery vascularized graft has led to excellent results, with a recently demonstrated 100% union rate with restoration of carpal parameters in 15 patients.[30]

WRIST ARTHRITIS

Optimal management of wrist arthritis remains challenging. Wrist denervation via anterior and posterior neurectomy is an attractive motion-preserving procedure that may offer durable results. In a retrospective case series of 100 wrists treated over a 21-year timeframe, 31% of patients required further procedures within 2 years, whereas the remaining 69% required no further procedure at an average follow-up of 6.75 years.[31] However, the highest failure rate was in SLAC or SNAC pattern wrists (43%), and for these patients, either a limited wrist fusion or a proximal row carpectomy (PRC) is often the reconstructive motion-preserving procedure of choice. When comparing these procedures, long-term nonrandomized studies have demonstrated slightly greater preservation of grip strength following 4-corner fusion and better motion preservation following PRC in patients younger than 45 years old.[32] However, large-scale analyses of the Veterans Health Administration[33] and Medicare claims databases[34] showed that patients undergoing 4-corner fusion required more secondary procedures and more conversions to wrist arthrodesis, respectively, suggesting that a PRC may be a more reliable procedure for most patients.

TENDON REPAIR

Flexor tenorrhaphy, particularly in zone 2, continues to push new boundaries in technique and philosophy. Strong, multicore suture repairs with 20% to 30% bunching at the repair site and judicious use of A2 and A4 pulley venting may obviate standard peripheral epitendinous sutures, as shown by the excellent outcomes of Giesen and colleagues[35] and Pan and colleagues.[36] Flexor tendon surgery performed with the WALANT technique allows observation of intraoperative active flexion-extension, and this careful assessment of repair site gapping enables true active motion protocols and decreased need for tenolysis. Pan and colleagues[36] evaluated their outcomes after a progressive evolution of surgical technique and rehabilitation protocol: from a 2-strand modified Kessler with a passive motion protocol, to 4- to 6-strand repairs with a true active motion protocol, to 6-strand repairs with an out-of-splint true active motion protocol, and found decreased rerupture rates (from 26% to 1.8% to 0%) and low rate of tenolysis (0%, 2%, 0%).[37] Novel suture designs and tendon coaptation devices may allow increased repair site strength, but it remains to be seen in vivo if the added strength is worth the added bulkiness to the repair.[38]

Although trigger digits are among the most common presenting complaint seen by most hand surgeons, nuances in optimal management continue to evolve. A corticosteroid injection often is the first-line treatment, but the choice between using a subsequent injection or proceeding to surgery often is predicated on patient desires and physician philosophy. Dardas and colleagues showed in their cohort of 292 consecutive second- or third-time injections that despite per-shot efficacy of long-term relief dropping to 39%, the median time to second or third injections was 371 and 407 days, respectfully, which is helpful to counsel patients. However, emerging evidence of the increased risk of infection following surgery of a recently injected site suggests caution. Matzon and colleagues showed in a large retrospective analysis of 2480 trigger finger releases that among the 1343 digits that had received a preoperative corticosteroid injection that there was an increased deep incisional infection risk from 0.1% to 0.8%, particularly among patients who had received their injection within 31 to 90 days preoperatively.[39] This group also examined the risk of both ipsilateral and contralateral corticosteroid injections for common indications at the time of clean, elective hand surgery for a separate diagnosis, and found an increased infection risk from 0.5% to 2.9% for injections ipsilateral to the procedure itself.[40] Although the exact mechanism for this susceptibility to infection remains uncertain, changes in injection patterns similar to that seen in the hip and knee arthroplasty literature with a greater delay between injection and surgery may decrease postoperative infection risk.

NERVE REPAIR

The recent publication of data from the RANGER trial shows promising advances in nerve repair surgery, particularly in the use of processed nerve allograft (PNA). For 624 peripheral nerve repairs, 82% meaningful recovery was achieved across sensory, mixed, and motor nerve repairs up to gaps of 70 mm[41], with similar results to autograft and better results than conduit reconstruction. In a separate publication specifically focusing on digital nerve repair with PNA versus conduit, a matched cohort comparison showed significantly better meaningful recovery in the PNA group for both short- (<14 mm) and long-gap (15–25 mm) repairs.[42] PNA appears to consistently provide similar outcomes as autograft reconstruction, without donor site morbidity. In the setting of proximal upper-extremity amputations, targeted muscle reinnervation (TMR) continues to show improvements in both residual limb pain (RLP) as well as phantom limb pain (PLP). Early TMR, in particular, improved the number of patients without PLP (24% to 62%) or RLP (36% to >50%) over delayed TMR.[43]

Both the diagnostic and therapeutic use of ultrasound in hand and upper-extremity surgery continues to evolve. In the evaluation of carpal tunnel syndrome (CTS), ultrasound was recently shown to have a lower false positive rate when compared with nerve conduction studies, making it potentially a more attractive option as a confirmatory diagnostic test.[44] It additionally can help discriminate severe CTS, particularly in patients younger than 65 years old or those with CTS-6 score greater than 12.[45] When patients with severe CTS present with thenar atrophy, it is customary to be cautious when predicting return of function; Garg and colleagues, however, evaluated patients with loss of opposition and palmar abduction and electrodiagnostic-confirmed severe CTS treated with open CTR and found that at 6 months all patients had greater tip/lateral/3-point pinch-and-grip strength, increased CMAP to the APB, and improved appearance on high-resolution MRI neurography, suggesting greater optimism for patients with preoperative atrophy.[46] Ultrasound additionally is helpful when evaluating ulnar nerve instability at the elbow, showing an 88% concordance between a preoperative ultrasound evaluation and intraoperative findings, compared with a 12% concordance between clinical examination and intraoperative findings.[47]

CLINICS CARE POINTS

- Multiple core strand zone 2 flexor tendon repairs with judicious A2 and A4 pulley venting, intraoperative assessment of active motion under WALANT, and true active motion rehabilitation protocols together are demonstrating excellent outcomes in the area formerly known as "no man's land."

- Processed nerve allograft, when used to bridge peripheral and digital nerve gaps, allows meaningful recovery similar to autograft and superior to conduit, even over long gaps.

DISCLOSURES

The author has no relevant financial disclosures.

REFERENCES

1. Stephens AR, Presson AP, McFarland MM, et al. Volar locked plating versus closed reduction and casting for acute, displaced distal radial fractures in the elderly: a systematic review and meta-analysis of randomized controlled trials. J Bone Joint Surg Am 2020;102(14):1280–8.
2. Angst F, Schwyzer H-K, Aeschlimann A, et al. Measures of adult shoulder function: disabilities of the arm, shoulder, and hand questionnaire (Dash) and its short version (Quickdash), shoulder pain and disability index (Spadi), american shoulder and elbow surgeons (Ases) society standardized shoulder assessment form, constant (Murley) score (Cs), simple shoulder test (Sst), oxford shoulder score (Oss), shoulder disability questionnaire (Sdq), and western ontario shoulder instability index(Wosi). Arthritis Care Res (Hoboken) 2011;63(Suppl 11): S174–88.
3. Landgren M, Teurneau V, Abramo A, et al. Intermediate-term outcome after distal radius fracture in patients with poor outcome at 1 year: a register study with a 2- to 12-year follow-up. J Hand Surg Am 2019;44(1):39–45.
4. Chung KC, Kim HM, Malay S, et al, WRIST Group. Predicting outcomes after distal radius fracture: a 24-center international clinical trial of older adults. J Hand Surg Am 2019;44(9):762–71.
5. Park MJ, Kim JP, Lee HI, et al. Is a short arm cast appropriate for stable distal radius fractures in patients older than 55 years? A randomized prospective multicentre study. J Hand Surg Eur Vol 2017; 42(5):487–92.
6. Landgren M, Abramo A, Geijer M, et al. Fragment-specific fixation versus volar locking plates in primarily nonreducible or secondarily redisplaced distal radius fractures: a randomized controlled study. J Hand Surg Am 2017;42(3):156–65.e1.
7. Galle SE, Harness NG, Hacquebord JH, et al. Complications of radial column plating of the distal radius. Hand (N Y) 2019;14(5):614–9.
8. Saving J, Enocson A, Ponzer S, et al. External fixation versus volar locking plate for unstable dorsally displaced distal radius fractures-a 3-year follow-up of a randomized controlled study. J Hand Surg Am 2019;44(1):18–26.
9. Costa ML, Achten J, Rangan A, et al. Percutaneous fixation with Kirschner wires versus volar locking-plate fixation in adults with dorsally displaced fracture of distal radius: five-year follow-up of a randomized controlled trial. Bone Joint J 2019;101-B(8):978–83.
10. Chung KC, Malay S, Shauver MJ, Wrist and Radius Injury Surgical Trial Group. The relationship between hand therapy and long-term outcomes after distal radius fracture in older adults: evidence from the randomized wrist and radius injury surgical trial. Plast Reconstr Surg 2019;144(2):230e–7e.
11. Substance Abuse and Mental Health Services Administration. Key substance use and mental health indicators in the United States: results from the 2018 National Survey on Drug Use and Health. 2019. Available at: https://www.samhsa.gov/data/sites/default/files/cbhsq-reports/NSDUHNationalFindingsReport2018/NSDUHNationalFindingsReport2018.pdf.
12. Bargon CA, Zale EL, Magidson J, et al. Factors associated with patients' perceived importance of opioid prescribing policies in an orthopedic hand surgery practice. J Hand Surg Am 2019;44(4):340.e1–8.
13. Stepan JG, Sacks HA, Lovecchio FC, et al. Opioid prescriber education and guidelines for ambulatory upper-extremity surgery: evaluation of an institutional protocol. J Hand Surg Am 2019;44(2):129–36.
14. Weinheimer K, Michelotti B, Silver J, et al. A prospective, randomized, double-blinded controlled trial comparing ibuprofen and acetaminophen

versus hydrocodone and acetaminophen for soft tissue hand procedures. J Hand Surg Am 2019; 44(5):387–93.

15. Dwyer CL, Soong M, Hunter A, et al. Prospective evaluation of an opioid reduction protocol in hand surgery. J Hand Surg Am 2018;43(6):516–22. e1.

16. Grandizio LC, Graham J, Klena JC. Current trends in walant surgery: a survey of american society for surgery of the hand members. J Hand Surg Glob Online 2020;2(4):186–90.

17. Aultman H, Roth CA, Curran J, et al. Prospective evaluation of surgical and anesthetic technique of carpal tunnel release in an orthopedic practice. J Hand Surg Am 2021;46(1):69.e1–7.

18. Patterson R. Carpometacarpal arthroplasty of the thumb. JBJS 1933;15(1):240–1.

19. Graham JG, Rivlin M, Ilyas AM. Unplanned early reoperation rate following thumb basal joint arthroplasty. J Hand Surg Glob Online 2020;2(1):21–4.

20. Ganhewa AD, Wu R, Chae MP, et al. Failure rates of base of thumb arthritis surgery: a systematic review. J Hand Surg Am 2019;44(9):728–41.e10.

21. DelSignore JL, Accardi KZ. Suture suspension arthroplasty technique for basal joint arthritis reconstruction. Tech Hand Up Extrem Surg 2009; 13(4):166–72.

22. Weiss A-PC, Kamal RN, Paci GM, et al. Suture suspension arthroplasty for the treatment of thumb carpometacarpal arthritis. J Hand Surg 2019;44(4): 296–303.

23. Rua T, Malhotra B, Vijayanathan S, et al. Clinical and cost implications of using immediate MRI in the management of patients with a suspected scaphoid fracture and negative radiographs results from the SMaRT trial. Bone Joint J 2019;101-B(8): 984–94.

24. Dias J, Brealey S, Cook L, et al. Surgical fixation compared with cast immobilisation for adults with a bicortical fracture of the scaphoid waist: the SWIFFT RCT. Health Technol Assess 2020;24(52): 1–234.

25. Clementson M, Jørgsholm P, Besjakov J, et al. Conservative treatment versus arthroscopic-assisted screw fixation of scaphoid waist fractures-a randomized trial with minimum 4-year follow-up. J Hand Surg 2015;40(7):1341–8.

26. Buijze GA, Goslings JC, Rhemrev SJ, et al, CAST Trial Collaboration. Cast immobilization with and without immobilization of the thumb for nondisplaced and minimally displaced scaphoid waist fractures: a multicenter, randomized, controlled trial. J Hand Surg Am 2014;39:621–7.

27. Grewal R, Suh N, MacDermid JC. The missed scaphoid fracture-outcomes of delayed cast treatment. J Wrist Surg 2015;4(4):278–83.

28. Mandaleson A, Tham SK, Lewis C, et al. Scaphoid fracture fixation in a nonunion model: a biomechanical study comparing 3 types of fixation. J Hand Surg 2018;43(3):221–8.

29. Rancy SK, Swanstrom MM, DiCarlo EF, et al. Success of scaphoid nonunion surgery is independent of proximal pole vascularity. J Hand Surg Eur Vol 2018;43(1):32–40.

30. Sommerkamp TG, Hastings H, Greenberg JA. Palmar radiocarpal artery vascularized bone graft for the unstable humpbacked scaphoid nonunion with an avascular proximal pole. J Hand Surg Am 2020;45(4):298–309.

31. O'Shaughnessy MA, Wagner ER, Berger RA, et al. Buying time: long-term results of wrist denervation and time to repeat surgery. Hand (N Y) 2019;14(5): 602–8.

32. Wagner ER, Werthel J-D, Elhassan BT, et al. Proximal row carpectomy and 4-corner arthrodesis in patients younger than age 45 years. J Hand Surg Am 2017;42(6):428–35.

33. Garcia BN, Lu C-C, Stephens AR, et al. Risk of total wrist arthrodesis or reoperation following 4-corner arthrodesis or proximal row carpectomy for stage-ii slac/snac arthritis: a propensity score analysis of 502 wrists. J Bone Joint Surg Am 2020;102(12): 1050–8.

34. Kay HF, Kang HP, Alluri RK, et al. Proximal row carpectomy versus 4-corner fusion: regional differences, incidence, and conversion to fusion: level 2 evidence. J Hand Surg 2018;43(9):S52–3.

35. Giesen T, Reissner L, Besmens I, et al. Flexor tendon repair in the hand with the M-Tang technique (Without peripheral sutures), pulley division, and early active motion. J Hand Surg Eur Vol 2018;43(5):474–9.

36. Pan ZJ, Xu YF, Pan L, et al. Zone 2 flexor tendon repairs using a tensioned strong core suture, sparse peripheral stitches and early active motion: results in 60 fingers. J Hand Surg Eur Vol 2019;44(4):361–6.

37. Pan ZJ, Pan L, Xu YF, et al. Outcomes of 200 digital flexor tendon repairs using updated protocols and 30 repairs using an old protocol: experience over 7 years. J Hand Surg Eur Vol 2020;45(1):56–63.

38. Wallace SJ, Mioton LM, Havey RM, et al. Biomechanical properties of a novel mesh suture in a cadaveric flexor tendon repair model. J Hand Surg Am 2019;44(3):208–15.

39. Matzon JL, Lebowitz C, Graham JG, et al. Risk of infection in trigger finger release surgery following corticosteroid injection. J Hand Surg Am 2020; 45(4):310–6.

40. Lutsky KF, Lucenti L, Banner L, et al. The effect of intraoperative corticosteroid injections on the risk of surgical site infections for hand procedures. J Hand Surg 2019;44(10):840–5.e5.

41. Safa B, Jain S, Desai MJ, et al. Peripheral nerve repair throughout the body with processed nerve allografts: results from a large multicenter study. Microsurgery 2020;40(5):527–37.

42. Leversedge FJ, Zoldos J, Nydick J, et al. A multi-center matched cohort study of processed nerve allograft and conduit in digital nerve reconstruction. J Hand Surg 2020;45(12):1148–56.

43. O'Brien AL, Jordan SW, West JM, et al. Targeted muscle reinnervation at the time of upper-extremity amputation for the treatment of pain severity and symptoms. J Hand Surg 2021;46(1):72.e1–10.

44. Fowler JR, Byrne K, Pan T, et al. False-positive rates for nerve conduction studies and ultrasound in patients without clinical signs and symptoms of carpal tunnel syndrome. J Hand Surg Am 2019;44(3): 181–5.

45. Nkrumah G, Blackburn AR, Goitz RJ, et al. Ultrasonography findings in severe carpal tunnel syndrome. Hand (N Y) 2020;15(1):64–8.

46. Garg B, Manhas V, Vardhan A, et al. Thumb opposition recovery following surgery for severe carpal tunnel syndrome: a clinical, radiological, and electrophysiological pilot study. J Hand Surg Am 2019;44(2):157.e1–5.

47. Rutter M, Grandizio LC, Malone WJ, et al. The use of preoperative dynamic ultrasound to predict ulnar nerve stability following in situ decompression for cubital tunnel syndrome. J Hand Surg Am 2019;44(1):35–8.

Shoulder and Elbow

Factors Influencing Appropriate Implant Selection and Position in Reverse Total Shoulder Arthroplasty

Jonathan Callegari, DO[a], Georges Haidamous, MD[b,c,d], Alexandre Lädermann, MD[e,f,g], Cameron Phillips, MD[a], Shane Tracy, PA-C[a], Patrick Denard, MD[a,h],*

KEYWORDS

- Reverse shoulder arthroplasty • Grammont • Lateralization • Neck-shaft angle • Glenoid version
- Onlay versus inlay • Reverse design

KEY POINTS

- The traditional Grammont design medialized and distalized the center of rotation, leading to improved deltoid torque and forward flexion, but less robust outcomes with rotation.
- The Grammont design had a high rate of scapular notching owing to lack of lateralization, eccentricity, and a higher neck-shaft angle.
- More lateralized designs lower the rate of scapular notching and lead to improved external rotation owing to increased tension on the remaining rotator cuff musculature.
- Range of motion outcomes may be optimized with more varus neck-shaft angles, larger glenospheres, inferior glenoid offset, and lateralization.
- Restoration of internal rotation remains an unsolved problem with reverse shoulder arthroplasty.

INTRODUCTION

The use of reverse shoulder arthroplasty (RSA) has increased dramatically in recent years as its indications have increased.[1] Although initially designed for the treatment of rotator cuff tear arthropathy, its indications have expanded to include primary glenohumeral arthritis, fractures, revision, instability, and others. In most patients, RSA leads to predictable pain relief and improvement in function. However, a subset of patients remains functionally limited following RSA.[2,3] In 1 study, up to 9% of patients were unimproved after RSA with continued pain and lower subjective outcomes.[4] Rauck and colleagues[5] found that among patients undergoing RSA, those with higher preoperative function had lower postoperative satisfaction scores, implying that RSA does not necessarily completely restore motion. Although outcomes

Funding: No industry funding was used for this study.
[a] Southern Oregon Orthopedics, 2780 East Barnett Road, Medford, OR 97504, USA; [b] University of South Florida Morsani College of Medicine, 12901 Bruce B Downs Boulevard, Tampa, FL 33612, USA; [c] Florida Orthopedic Institute, 13020 Telecom Pkwy N, Temple Terrace, FL 33637, USA; [d] Foundation for Orthopedic Research and Education, Tampa, FL, USA; [e] Division of Orthopaedics and Trauma Surgery, La Tour Hospital, Av J.-D. Maillard 3, Meyrin CH-1217, Switzerland; [f] Faculty of Medicine, University of Geneva, Rue Michel-Servet 1, Geneva 4 1211, Switzerland; [g] Division of Orthopaedics and Trauma Surgery, Department of Surgery, Geneva University Hospitals, Rue Gabrielle-Perret-Gentil 4, Geneva 14 1211, Switzerland; [h] Department of Orthopaedics and Rehabilitation, Oregon Health and Science University, Portland, OR, USA
* Corresponding author. Southern Oregon Orthopedics, 2780 East Barnett Road, Medford, OR 97504.
E-mail address: pjdenard@gmail.com

may be partially influenced by indication, this also may relate to design factors and implant positioning.

The initial Grammont prosthesis design was created to offer improved biomechanical advantages to address the failures at the time with previous RSA designs. A medialized center of rotation (placed on the face of the glenoid) reduced torque seen by the glenoid component at the point of fixation. It was also proposed that moving the center of rotation medially and distally increased the deltoid lever arm and increased deltoid tension.[6] This design had excellent restoration of forward flexion but led to little improvement in rotation. It also presented a high rate of scapular notching.[7] These problems led to a variety of modifications, particularly increased glenoid lateralization and more anatomic neck-shaft angle of the humeral component. Although the central goal remains achieving good fixation and restoring glenohumeral stability, modern RSA designs are highly varied on both the humerus and the glenoid. Moreover, component position can vary substantially in RSA. The purpose of this review is to provide an in-depth examination of how humeral and glenoid component design as well as implant position impacts functional outcomes following RSA.

HUMERAL FACTORS

Humeral factors that may influence functional outcome and complication profile include the neck-shaft angle, inlay versus onlay epiphyseal component, humeral lateralization, polyethylene design, and component version.

Neck-Shaft Angle

The original Grammont design was characterized by a nonanatomic 155° neck-shaft angle. More modern designs have moved to either a 145° or 135° neck-shaft angle. This modification has been validated in computer-modeling studies as well as in clinical studies.[8–11]

Gutierrez and colleagues[12,13] examined the hierarchy of factors influencing range of motion (ROM) in a computer simulation and determined that the neck-shaft angle had the single biggest impact on reducing the adduction deficit (reducing notching). They recommended a more anatomic neck-shaft angle, such as 135°. Likewise, Lädermann and colleagues[14] performed a 3-dimensional (3D) computer-modeling study assessing the differences in ROM between a traditional Grammont inlay prosthesis and various configurations of onlay

prostheses. They found that a reduced neck-shaft angle (135° or 145°) led to a dramatic improvement in adduction as well as extension and external rotation with the arm at the side. Forward flexion was unchanged, and a small decrease in abduction was observed. This study, along with other studies, also demonstrated that abduction decreases as humeral inclination becomes more anatomic.[10] Jeon and colleagues[15] also performed a 3D computer model examining the combined effects of neck-shaft angle and retroversion of the humeral component. Decreasing the neck-shaft angle to 135° resulted in improved total horizontal ROM with an improved adduction deficit compared with a 155° prosthesis. The amount of humeral retrotorsion was inversely proportional to internal rotation.[16] In a 3D computer templating model, Werner and colleagues[17] found that a 135° neck-shaft angle (compared with 145°) had a larger impingement-free ROM with improved adduction, extension, and external rotation with the arm at the side.[18] In a virtual shoulder model, Virani and colleagues[19] examined the effects of implant-related factors on impingement-free ROM. They found that the neck-shaft angle was the most predictive factor in determining abduction and forward elevation. The 130° prosthesis resulted in significantly fewer impingements compared with a 150° prosthesis (**Fig. 1**).

Clinically, decreasing the neck-shaft angle may provide benefits without sacrificing ROM. Gobezie and colleagues[20] performed a randomized controlled trial of RSA for rotator cuff arthropathy comparing 135° to a 155° neck-shaft angles with a neutral glenosphere. They found that although there were no significant differences in ROM, the rate of scapular notching was decreased with the 135° prosthesis (21% vs 58%). In a systematic review, Erickson and colleagues[21] found that a 135° prosthesis had a lowered rate of scapular notching (2.8%) compared with a 155° prosthesis (16.8%). Oh and colleagues[22] performed a cadaveric study examining the effects of various neck-shaft angles on humeral impingement and ROM. They found that decreasing the neck-shaft angle led to a greater arc of ROM before impingement and small improvements in external rotation compared with a 155° prosthesis.[23]

Inlay Versus Onlay Prosthesis

There are 2 main types of humeral cups: an inlay and an onlay. The classic Grammont design featured a straight stem with an inlay humeral cup. In this design, a portion of the proximal humerus is reamed out so that the articulating

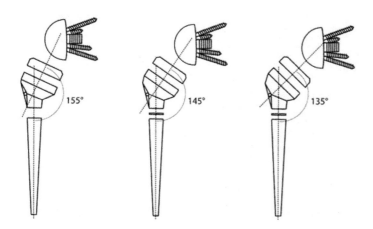

Fig. 1. Humeral implant inclination angles. (*From* Oh JH, Shin SJ, McGarry MH, et al. Biomechanical effects of humeral neck-shaft angle and subscapularis integrity in reverse total shoulder arthroplasty. J Shoulder Elbow Surg 2014;23(8):1093; with permission.)

surface is below the humeral cut. In an onlay design, the articulation is placed on top of the humeral cut surface. The latter was adopted as a way to make an anatomic stem convertible to an RSA (by placing an articulating adaptor on top of the same humeral cut surface that could be used for an anatomic cut). This modification leads to biomechanical and anatomic consequences. Because the articulation of an onlay occurs above the humeral cut level, it leads to both lateralization and distalization of the humerus relative to the center of rotation.[24]

Proponents of this design type argue that humeral lateralization increases the deltoid lever arm and thus function via a deltoid "wrapping" effect.[2] Beltrame and colleagues[24] reported that an onlay 145° design provided increased improvement in adduction, external rotation, and extension compared with a 155° inlay prosthesis. There was no significant difference in internal rotation between the 2 groups. On the other hand, distalization may increase the risk of neurologic injury[25–27] and scapular spine fracture.[28,29] In a prospective study, Lowe and colleagues[30] found that RSA with a lateralized glenosphere and a 135° inlay cup decreased arm lengthening compared with the traditional Grammont design and lowered the risk of neurologic injury. LeDuc and colleagues[31] demonstrated that an onlay prosthesis led to an increased rate of acromial stress fractures compared with an inlay prosthesis.[32] Haidamous and colleagues[28] compared 3 different RSA prostheses (2 inlay and 1 onlay) and found a significantly increased risk of scapular spine fractures with an onlay prosthesis compared with inlay designs (11.9% vs 4.7%). Notably, the risk of scapular spine fracture was associated with increased distalization but not lateralization (**Fig. 2**).

Lateralization on the Humeral Side

The concept of lateralization developed to decrease the traditionally high rate of scapular notching and impingement with the Grammont inlay (medialized) design. Lateralization on the humeral side can be achieved by switching to an onlay prosthesis or using a lower neck-shaft angle. With an onlay prosthesis, the polyethylene is placed more medial (promoting lateralization) and also lateralizes the stem away from the glenosphere compared with an inlay prosthesis. These factors have important implications in improving rotator cuff tension and the deltoid moment arm.[33,34] Lateralization has been theorized to increase torque at the glenoid interface and potentially lead to loosening.[35] Giles and colleagues[36] demonstrated that with increasing humeral lateralization up to 10 mm, the force required from the deltoid for abduction lowered from 68% to 65% body weight, which may help counteract increasing joint loading occurring with glenoid-based lateralization. A lateralized humeral component combined with a decreased neck-shaft angle has been shown to decrease scapular notching rates in comparison to a medialized humeral design.[14] Merolla and colleagues[37] performed a retrospective cohort study comparing a Grammont design versus a curved onlay design and found a lower rate of scapular notching and significant improvement in external rotation. A risk with increasing lateralization is deltoid-related pain owing to increased soft tissue tension.[28,38]

Torsion

Historically, it was recommended that the Grammont prosthesis be placed in 0° of retrotorsion (torsion is used to describe the position of the humeral stem, whereas version is used to describe the position of the glenosphere). This

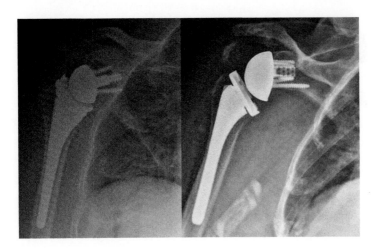

Fig. 2. Comparison of inlay versus onlay reverse arthroplasty stems.

recommendation was an effort to compensate for the lack of postoperative internal rotation that was seen with this design. Many investigators now recommend a more anatomic torsion of 20° to 30°. Kontaxis and colleagues[39] compared simulated activities of daily living with different versions of a 135° onlay humeral component. Increasing retrotorsion was associated with a greater ROM but with increased impingement between the coracoid and the greater tuberosity. Antetorsion was associated with impingement and scapular notching as well as reduced ROM.[40,41] Boileau and colleagues[7] demonstrated that increasing retrotorsion results in increased external rotation at the expense of an internal rotation deficit.

Stephenson and colleagues[42] performed a cadaveric study examining retrotorsion on ROM outcomes and impingement with an onlay system. In this study, the overall arc of motion was constant with regards to torsion. Increasing humeral retrotorsion improved external rotation at the cost of internal rotation before impingement. They suggested 20° to 40° of retrotorsion to maximize impingement-free ROM. However, other studies, such as those performed by Aleem and colleagues[43] and Rhee and colleagues,[44] demonstrated no improved functional outcomes in regards to rotation ROM based on the amount of humeral torsion at minimum 2-year follow-up.

Berhouet and colleagues[45] examined the effect of humeral retrotorsion and glenosphere size on scapular notching in a cadaveric study. Using an onlay system, they observed that impingement and scapular notching occurred the earliest with a smaller glenosphere sized (36 mm) and latest with a larger glenosphere (42 mm) and lateralization. This combination

also improved adduction ROM. They also noticed an effect of humeral retrotorsion: 10° to 20° produced less impingement than higher levels of humeral retrotorsion without a significant effect on overall abduction ROM.

Polyethylene

Stability of the prosthesis depends on the contact area between the glenosphere and polyethylene. Minimal contact results in high mobility but less stability, whereas maximum contact results in greater stability with a more constrained nature.[13] Similar to total hip arthroplasty, the nature of a more constrained humeral insert carries a risk of increased wear and aseptic loosening.[46]

Reducing the depth of the polyethylene cup may increase motion and limit impingement. DeWilde and colleagues[47] found that decreasing the polyethylene depth by 3 mm increased ROM by 12°. As Lädermann and colleagues[14] noted, based on impingement between the humeral cup and the scapular neck in the position of adduction, extension, and neutral rotation, 1 consideration is to use polyethylene cups with a notch between 3 and 9 o'clock. However, no studies have demonstrated this benefit.

GLENOID FACTORS

Glenoid factors that may influence ROM include lateralization, glenosphere size, and glenosphere position.

Lateralization on the Glenoid Side

Before the inception of Grammont's design, RSA failed largely because of glenoid baseplate loosening. By medializing the center of rotation, this problem was solved at the time. However, this came at the expense of a high rate of scapular notching ranging from 5% to 51%.[48] In addition to mechanical impingement (notching), poor rotation was also obtained because the remaining rotator cuff was medialized and not under appropriate tension.[6] Modern designs provide enhanced glenoid-sided fixation and allow lateralization. Such lateralization may lower the rate of scapular notching and provide improved rotational motion.[49,50] Lädermann and colleagues[51,52] studied 3D computer models with multiple constructs and found that glenoid-sided lateralization achieved greater ROM in all movements. Lateralization also leads to an improvement in posterior deltoid fiber recruitment, which may contribute to increased external rotation.[53] In the study by Virani and colleagues,[19] they found that a construct with 10 mm of glenosphere lateralization provided the greatest impingement-free ROM of all constructs and was the second most important factor in predicting ROM in abduction and forward elevation. The 10-mm lateralized models also had lower rates of scapular impingement compared with less-lateralized models.

Two options are available for lateralization: bony and metallic. Although there are subtle differences, both techniques are supported clinically. Bony lateralization or a bony increase offset (BIO)-RSA construct is created by placing bone beneath the baseplate, which relies on the graft integrating to the baseplate and the glenoid. On the other hand, metallic lateralization via the baseplate or glenosphere requires integration of only 1 surface. Denard and colleagues[54] performed a computation finite element analysis (FEA) on the effects of lateralization in RSA. Four different glenoid models were used: standard glenosphere (36 mm) without lateralization, a glenosphere with bone graft, a glenosphere with a lateralized baseplate, and a lateralized glenosphere. Displacement during the FEA analysis was lower with metallic augmentation (lateralized glenosphere or baseplate). Notably, the bony model exceeded theoretic levels for osseous integration between 5 and 10 mm. Athwal and colleagues[55] studied the use of standard Grammont-style RSA versus a BIO-RSA and found a lower scapular notching rate (40% vs 75% for standard) without a significant change in ROM (Fig. 3).

Theoretically, lateralization may have a mechanical tradeoff because it decreases the moment arm of the deltoid and therefore its efficiency with ROM. With increasing lateralization there is also an increase in stress at the glenoid-baseplate interface, which may theoretically lead to loosening.[35] Hettrich and colleagues[35]

performed a biomechanical model in which they compared ROM through finite element analysis with an RSA system in different combinations of medialization and lateralization. The medialized system was compared to reflect the typical medialized wear pattern usually seen in rotator cuff arthropathy and compared with a lateralized system with BIO-RSA grafts of different thickness. They found that all lateralized glenospheres resulted in larger impingement-free ROM compared with the medialized model with the 2.5-mm model achieving the largest impingement-free ROM. Increasing lateralization required a larger deltoid force to result in abduction: for every 1 mm of lateralization achieved, there was a 6.8% difference in deltoid force required for ROM. However, it is important to note that the concept of lateralization is in comparison to Grammont's original design and a "lateralized" design is still medialized compared with the native glenohumeral joint.[40]

Glenosphere Size

The advantage of increasing glenosphere size is to offer a greater arc of motion with increased stability.[6] Berhouet and colleagues[45] demonstrated that larger glenospheres increase ROM and reduce impingement. In a retrospective analysis with a 155° inlay prosthesis, Muller and colleagues[56,57] found that a larger glenosphere size (44 vs 36 mm) resulted in approximately 12° improvement in external rotation. Haidamous and colleagues[2] suggested that a glenosphere size of 39 mm was associated with a 9.2 times increased chance of an excellent outcome. In their computer simulation model, Virani and colleagues[19] found that a 42-mm glenosphere provided the greatest arc of ROM compared with smaller glenospheres and was the second most predictive factor for rotational ROM. However, larger glenospheres may have the consequence of increasing volumetric polyethylene wear.[58] In addition, oversizing the glenoid may have consequences such as overstuffing.[59] In other words, there is likely an ideal glenosphere size for each patient, but currently patient-specific guidelines for glenosphere size are lacking.

Glenosphere Positioning

Positioning of the glenosphere in space may affect ROM and impingement, whereas lateralization remains unaffected. Glenosphere positioning can be manipulated both in the cranial-caudal directions and with superior-inferior tilt.

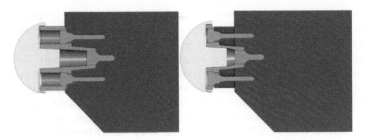

Fig. 3. Glenoid lateralization options: metallic versus BIO-RSA. (*From* Denard PJ, Lederman E, Parsons BO, et al. Finite element analysis of glenoid-sided lateralization in reverse shoulder arthroplasty. J Orthop Res 2017;35(7):1549; with permission.)

It is clear today that superior tilt of the glenosphere results in loosening and ultimate failure.[60] Many studies have attempted to find a benefit with inferior glenoid tilt, but few have been successful. Some biomechanical studies suggest that 10° of inferior tilt provides the greatest impingement-free arc of ROM.[61] This degree of inferior tilt, however, has not been proven clinically. Edwards and colleagues[62] completed a randomized controlled trial to compare glenoids with neutral inclination to those with 10° inferior tilt and found no difference in outcomes or scapular notching rates.

An eccentric position of the glenosphere, with overhang inferiorly, has been shown to improve adduction and abduction.[12,63] Inferior overhang of the glenosphere may provide up to 39° of additional adduction without impingement.[47] Haidamous and colleagues[2] examined the relationship between radiographic parameters and outcomes after RSA. The only radiographic factor associated with an excellent outcome was inferior glenoid offset. They recommended a mean inferior overhang of 3.1 mm beyond the inferior glenoid. In a 3D computed tomography simulator study, Kolmodin and colleagues[9] found that an average of 3.4 mm of inferior translation of the baseplate was necessary to avoid scapular impingement. Virani and colleagues[19] found that, of all constructs tested, all models with inferior glenosphere placement had no adduction deficit nor impingement with the arm at the side. They also found that when changing the glenosphere from a neutral to an inferior position there was a 32% increase in rotation ROM. There is, however, a limit to the amount of acceptable overhang without leading to baseplate loosening and the negative effects of arm lengthening[6,64] (**Fig. 4**).

Using a 145° inlay design, Lädermann and colleagues[51] reported that an eccentric (2 mm inferior) 36-mm glenosphere provided better impingement-free ROM compared with a neutral 36-mm, 42-mm, or 36-mm sphere with 10-mm lateralization or 10° of tilt while limiting scapular notching.

THE IDEAL CONSTRUCT

The current available literature suggests the ideal construct to improve ROM and reduce impingement is a 135° neck-shaft angle humeral component placed in neutral or slight retrotorsion with a large glenosphere with inferior overhang and up to 10 mm of baseplate lateralization.[19,65–67] However, much of these recommendations are based on computer modeling, and further clinical studies are required. Computer-modeling studies are limited in their ability to account for soft tissue tension and muscle quality. In the authors' opinion, for instance, lateralization can partially be based off of age and strength with higher degrees of lateralization (ie, 6–8 mm) used in younger patients and more moderate degrees of lateralization (ie, 4 mm) for patients over the age of 80 based on the increased deltoid force requirements of lateralized implants.

Gaining internal rotation remained a problem after Grammont-style RSA. Boileau and colleagues[7] reported that mean internal rotation was to the first sacral vertebra postoperatively and rarely improved after RSA, which was attributed to the medialized design of the Grammont style prosthesis. With modern prostheses, internal rotation may be limited by lateralization, larger glenospheres, and humeral stem retrotorsion.[68,69] Functional internal rotation is typically worse after RSA compared with TSA.[70] To this day, gaining internal rotation remains a problem after RSA.[7,43]

In the future, there is a need to move to more patient-specific guidelines in order to optimize outcomes after RSA. Some studies suggest patient-specific guides or 3D preoperative planning improves component positioning during RSA.[53,67,71,72] Furthermore, as postoperative ROM is related to hundreds of variables with thousands of possible combinations, artificial intelligence may hold promise in determining the best preoperative theoretic design and positioning.

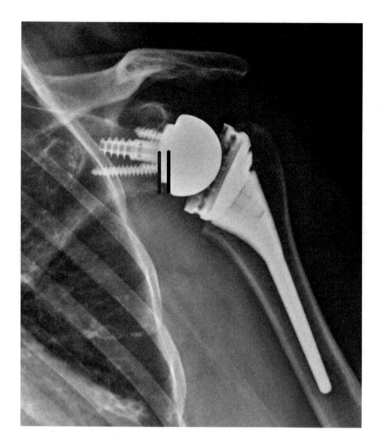

Fig. 4. Inferior glenoid offset calculated as the distance from the center of the glenoid to the inferior border of the glenosphere (*black line*) minus the distance from the center of the glenosphere to the inferior border of the scapular neck (*blue line*).

SUMMARY

Statistically, outcomes after RSA are great; however, a subset of patients may not achieve satisfactory outcome measures. Specifically, internal rotation does not improve as consistently as forward elevation and external rotation. Certain design choices may influence ROM outcomes following RSA.

CLINICS CARE POINTS

- Inferior glenosphere overhang is recommended to avoid impingement.
- Larger glenospheres provide a greater impingement-free range of motion.
- Superior tilt of the glenosphere leads to ultimate failure of the implant.
- Lateralization improves impingement-free ROM.
- There is an increased risk of neurologic injuries and acromial stress fractures with an onlay prosthesis compared with an inlay prosthesis.

DISCLOSURE

Dr P. Denard: consultant, research support, and royalties, Arthrex; paid speakers bureau, Pacira, Inc. Dr A. Lädermann: paid consultant, Arthrex, Wright, and Medacta and royalties, Wright. Dr J. Callegari, Dr G. Haidamous, Dr C. Phillips, and Mr S. Tracy, their immediate family, and any research foundation with which they are affiliated have not received any financial payments or other benefits from any commercial entity related to the subject of this article.

REFERENCES

1. Best M, Azul K, Wilckens J, et al. Increasing Incidence of primary reverse and anatomic total shoulder arthroplasty in the United States. J Shoulder Elbow Surg 2020. https://doi.org/10.1016/j.jse.2020.08.010.

2. Haidamous G, Lädermann A, Hartzler R, et al. Radiographic parameters associated with excellent versus poor range of motion outcomes following reverse shoulder arthroplasty. Shoulder Elbow 2020;0(0):1–9.

3. Hamilton MA, Diep P, Roche C, et al. Effect of reverse shoulder design philosophy on muscle moment arms. J Orthop Res 2015;33(4):605–13.

4. Parsons M, Routman HD, Roche CP, et al. Patient-reported outcomes of reverse total shoulder arthroplasty: a comparative risk factor analysis of improved versus unimproved cases. J Shoulder Elbow Surg Open Access 2019;3(3):174–8.

5. Rauck RC, Ruzbarsky JJ, Swarup I, et al. Predictors of patient satisfaction after reverse shoulder arthroplasty. J Shoulder Elbow Surg 2020;29(3):e67–74.

6. Middernacht B, Van Tongel A, DeWilde L. A critical review on prosthetic features available for reversed total shoulder arthroplasty. Biomed Res Int 2016; 2016:3256931.

7. Boileau P, Watkinson DJ, Hatzidakis AM, et al. Grammont reverse prosthesis: design, rationale, and biomechanics. J Shoulder Elbow Surg 2005; 14(1 suppl S):147S–61S.

8. Gutiérrez S, Comiskey C, Luo ZP, et al. Range of impingement-free abduction and adduction deficit after reverse shoulder arthroplasty. J Bone Joint Surg Am 2008;90(12):2606–15.

9. Kolmodin J, Davidson IU, Jun BJ, et al. Scapular notching after reverse total shoulder arthroplasty: prediction using patient-specific osseous anatomy, implant location, and shoulder motion. J Bone Joint Surg Am 2018;100(13):1095–103.

10. Lädermann A, Denard P, Boileau P. Effect of humeral stem design on humeral position and range of motion in reverse shoulder arthroplasty. Int Orthop 2015;39(11):2205–13.

11. Langohr G, Giles J, Athwal G, et al. The effect of glenosphere diameter in reverse shoulder arthroplasty on muscle force, joint load, and range of motion. J Shoulder Elbow Surg 2015;24(6):972–9.

12. Gutierrez S, Levy J, Frankle M, et al. Evaluation of abduction range of motion and avoidance of inferior scapular impingement in a reverse shoulder model. J Shoulder Elbow Surg 2008;17(4):608–15.

13. Gutierrez S, Luo Z, Levy J, et al. Arc of motion and socket depth in reverse shoulder arthroplasty implants. Clin Biomech 2009;24(6):473–9.

14. Lädermann A, Geuorguiev B, Charbonnier C. Scapular notching on kinematic simulated range of motion after reverse shoulder arthroplasty is not the result of impingement in adduction. Medicine 2015;94(38):e1615.

15. Jeon BK, Panchal K, Ji JH, et al. Combined effect of change in humeral neck-shaft angle and retroversion on shoulder range of motion in reverse total shoulder arthroplasty—a simulation study. Clin Biomech 2016;31:12–9.

16. Keener JD, Chalmers PN, Yamaguchi K. The humeral implant in shoulder arthroplasty. J Am Acad Orthop Surg 2017;25(6):427–38.

17. Werner BS, Chaoui J, Walch G. The influence of humeral neck shaft angle and glenoid lateralization on range of motion in reverse shoulder arthroplasty. J Shoulder Elbow Surg 2017;26(10):1726–31.

18. Werthel JD, Walch G, Vegehan E, et al. Lateralization in reverse shoulder arthroplasty: a descriptive analysis of different implants in current practice. Int Orthop 2019;43(10):2349–60.

19. Virani N, Cabezas A, Gutierrez S, et al. Reverse shoulder arthroplasty components and surgical techniques that restore glenohumeral motion. J Shoulder Elbow Surg 2013;22:179–87.

20. Gobezie R, Shishani Y, Lederman E, et al. Can a functional difference be detected in reverse arthroplasty with 135° versus 155° prosthesis for the treatment of rotator cuff arthropathy: a prospective randomized study. J Shoulder Elbow Surg 2019; 28(5):813–8.

21. Erickson BJ, Frank RM, Harris JD, et al. The influence of humeral head inclination in reverse total shoulder arthroplasty: a systematic review. J Shoulder Elbow Surg 2015;24(6):988–93.

22. Oh JH, Shin SJ, McGarry M, et al. Biomechanical effects of humeral neck-shaft angle and subscapularis integrity in reverse total shoulder arthroplasty. J Shoulder Elbow Surg 2014;23(8):1091–8.

23. Parry S, Stachler S, Mahylis J. Lateralization in reverse shoulder arthroplasty: a review. J Orthop 2020;22:64–7.

24. Beltrame A, Di Benedetto P, Cicuto C, et al. Onlay versus inlay humeral stem in reverse shoulder arthroplasty (RSA): clinical and biomechanical study. Acta Biomed 2019;90(Suppl 12):54–63.

25. Kim HJ, Kwon TY, Jeon YS, et al. Neurologic deficit after reverse total shoulder arthroplasty: correlation with distalization. J Shoulder Elbow Surg 2020; 29(6):1096–103.

26. Lädermann A, Lübbeke A, Mélis B, et al. Prevalence of neurologic lesions after total shoulder arthroplasty. J Bone Joint Surg Am 2011;93(14):1288–93.

27. Lädermann A, Tay E, Collin P, et al. Effect of critical shoulder angle, glenoid lateralization, and humeral inclination on range of movement in reverse shoulder arthroplasty. Bone Joint Res 2019;3(8):378–86.

28. Haidamous G, Lädermann A, Frankle M, et al. The risk of postoperative scapular spine fracture following reverse shoulder arthroplasty is increased with an onlay humeral stem. J Shoulder Elbow Surg 2020;29(12):2556–63.

29. Wong M, Langohr D, Athwal G, et al. Implant positioning in reverse shoulder arthroplasty has an impact on acromial stresses. J Shoulder Elbow Surg 2016;25(11):1889–95.

30. Lowe JT, Lawler SM, Testa EJ, et al. Lateralization of the glenosphere in reverse shoulder arthroplasty decreases arm lengthening and demonstrates comparable risk of nerve injury compared with anatomic arthroplasty: a prospective cohort study. J Shoulder Elbow Surg 2018;27(10):1845–51.

31. LeDuc R, Salazar D, Garbis N. Incidence of postoperative acromial fractures with onlay vs inlay

reverse shoulder arthroplasty. J Shoulder Elbow Surg 2019;28(6):e206.

32. Levigne C, Boileau P, Favard L, et al. Scapular notching in reverse shoulder arthroplasty. J Shoulder Elbow Surg 2008;17(6):925–35.

33. Hansen M, Routman H. The biomechanics of current reverse shoulder replacement options. Ann Joint 2019;4:17.

34. Hasan S, Levy J, Leitze Z, et al. Reverse shoulder prosthesis with a lateralized glenosphere: early results of a prospective multicenter study stratified by diagnosis. J Shoulder Elbow Surg 2019;3:1–9.

35. Hettrich C, Permeswaran V, Goetz J, et al. Mechanical tradeoffs associated with glenosphere lateralization in reverse shoulder arthroplasty. J Shoulder Elbow Surg 2015;24(11):1774–81.

36. Giles JW, Langohr GD, Johnson JA, et al. Implant design variations in reverse total shoulder arthroplasty influence the required deltoid force and resultant joint load. Clin Orthop Relat Res 2015; 473(11):3615–26.

37. Merolla G, Walch G, Ascione F, et al. Grammont humeral design versus onlay curved-stem reverse shoulder arthroplasty: comparison of clinical and radiographic outcomes with minimum 2-year follow-up. J Shoulder Elbow Surg 2018;27(4): 701–10.

38. Chan K, Langohr G, Mahaffy M, et al. Does humeral component lateralization in reverse shoulder arthroplasty affect rotator cuff torque? Evaluation in a cadaver model. Clin Orthop Relat Res 2017; 475(10):2564–71.

39. Kontaxis A, Chen X, Berhouet J, et al. Humeral version in reverse shoulder arthroplasty affects impingement in activities of daily living. J Shoulder Elbow Surg 2017;26:1073–82.

40. Roche CP, Diep P, Hamilton M, et al. Impact of inferior glenoid tilt, humeral retroversion, bone grafting, and design parameters on muscle length and deltoid wrapping in reverse shoulder arthroplasty. Bull Hosp Jt Dis 2013;71(4):284–93.

41. Sheth U, Saltzman M. Reverse total shoulder arthroplasty: implant design considerations. Curr Rev Musculoskelet Med 2019;12:554–61.

42. Stephenson DR, Oh JH, McGarry MH, et al. Effect of humeral component version on impingement in reverse total shoulder arthroplasty. J Shoulder Elbow Surg 2011;20(4):652–8.

43. Aleem AW, Feeley BT, Austin LS, et al. Effect of humeral component version on outcomes in reverse shoulder arthroplasty. Orthopedics 2017;40(3): 179–86.

44. Rhee YG, Cho NS, Moon SC. Effects of humeral component retroversion on functional outcomes in reverse total shoulder arthroplasty for cuff tear arthropathy. J Shoulder Elbow Surg 2015;24(10): 1574–81.

45. Berhouet J, Garaud P, Favard L. Evaluation of the role of glenosphere design and humeral component retroversion in avoiding scapular notching during reverse shoulder arthroplasty. J Shoulder Elbow Surg 2014;23(2):151–8.

46. Carpenter S, Pinkas D, Newton M, et al. Wear rates of retentive versus nonretentive reverse total shoulder arthroplasty liners in an in vitro wear simulation. J Shoulder Elbow Surg 2015;24(9):1372–9.

47. DeWilde L, Poncet D, Middernacht B, et al. Prosthetic overhang is the most effective way to prevent scapular conflict in a reverse total shoulder prosthesis. Acta Orthop 2010;6:719–26.

48. Alentorn-Geli E, Samitier G, Torrens C, et al. Reverse shoulder arthroplasty. Part 2: systematic review of reoperations, revisions, problems, and complications. Int J Shoulder Surg 2015;9:60–7.

49. Cuff D, Clark R, Pupello D, et al. Reverse shoulder arthroplasty for the treatment of rotator cuff deficiency: a concise follow-up, at a minimum of five years, of a previous report. J Bone Joint Surg Am 2012;94(21):1996–2000.

50. Cuff D, Pupello D, Santoni B, et al. Reverse shoulder arthroplasty for the treatment of rotator cuff deficiency: a concise follow-up, at a minimum of 10 years, of previous reports. J Bone Joint Surg Am 2017;99(22):1895–9.

51. Lädermann A, Denard P, Collin P, et al. Effect of humeral stem and glenosphere designs on range of motion and muscle length in reverse shoulder arthroplasty. Int Orthop 2020;44:519–30.

52. Lädermann A, Denard P, Boileau P. What is the best glenoid configuration in onlay reverse shoulder arthroplasty? Int Orthop 2018;42:1339–46.

53. Iannotti JP, Weiner S, Rodriguez E, et al. Three-dimensional imaging and templating improve glenoid implant positioning. J Bone Joint Surg Am 2015;97(8):651–8.

54. Denard P, Lederman E, Parsons B, et al. Finite-element analysis of glenoid-sided lateralization in reverse shoulder arthroplasty. J Orthop Res 2016; 35(7):1548–55.

55. Athwal GS, MacDermid JC, Reddy KM, et al. Does bony increased-offset reverse shoulder arthroplasty decrease scapular notching? J Shoulder Elbow Surg 2015;24(3):468–73.

56. Muller A, Born M, Jung C, et al. Glenosphere size in reverse shoulder arthroplasty: is larger better for external rotation and abduction strength? J Shoulder Elbow Surg 2018;27:44–52.

57. Nelson R, Lowe JT, Lawler SM, et al. Lateralized center of rotation and lower neck-shaft angle are associated with lower rates of scapular notching and heterotopic ossification and improved pain for reverse shoulder arthroplasty at 1 year. Orthopedics 2018;41(4):230–6.

58. Haggart J, Newton M, Hartner S, et al. Neer Award 2017: wear rates of 32-mm and 40-mm glenospheres in a reverse total shoulder arthroplasty wear simulation model. J Shoulder Elbow Surg 2017;6:2029–37.

59. Matsuki K, King J, Wright T, et al. Outcomes of reverse shoulder arthroplasty in small- and large-stature patients. J Shoulder Elbow Surg 2018; 27(5):808–15.

60. Randelli P, Randelli F, Arrigoni P, et al. Optimal glenoid component inclination in reverse shoulder arthroplasty. How to improve stability. Musculoskelet Surg 2014;98(Suppl 1):15–8.

61. Gutierrez S, Walker M, Willis M, et al. Effects of tilt and glenosphere eccentricity on baseplate/bone interface forces in a computational model, validated by a mechanical model, of reverse shoulder arthroplasty. J Shoulder Elbow Surg 2011;20(5): 641–6.

62. Edwards T, Trappey G, Riley C, et al. Inferior tilt of the glenoid component does not decrease scapular notching in reverse shoulder arthroplasty: results of a prospective randomized study. J Shoulder Elbow Surg 2012;21(5):641–6.

63. Nyffeler R, Werner C, Gerber C. Biomechanical relevance of glenoid component positioning in the reverse Delta III total shoulder prosthesis. J Shoulder Elbow Surg 2005;14(5):524–8.

64. Friedman R, Barcel D, Eichinger J. Scapular notching in reverse total shoulder arthroplasty. J ASOS 2019;27(6):200–9.

65. Keener J, Patterson B, Orvets N, et al. Optimizing reverse shoulder arthroplasty component position in the setting of advanced arthritis with posterior glenoid erosion: a computer-enhance range of motion analysis. J Shoulder Elbow Surg 2018;27: 339–49.

66. Kerrigan A, Reeves J, Langohr D, et al. Reverse shoulder arthroplasty glenoid lateralization influences scapular spine strains. Shoulder Elbow 2020;1–10.

67. Walch G, Vezeridis PS, Boileau P, et al. Three-dimensional planning and use of patient-specific guides improve glenoid component position: an in vitro study. J Shoulder Elbow Surg 2015;24(2): 302–9.

68. Berhouet J, Garaud P, Favard L. Influence of glenoid component design and humeral component retroversion on internal and external rotation in reverse shoulder arthroplasty: a cadaver study. Orthop Traumatol Surg Res 2013;99(8):887–94.

69. Berhouet J, Kontaxis A, Gulotta L, et al. Effects of the humeral tray component positioning for onlay reverse shoulder arthroplasty design: a biomechanical analysis. J Shoulder Elbow Surg 2015;24(4): 569–77.

70. Triplet JJ, Everding NG, Levy JC, et al. Functional internal rotation after shoulder arthroplasty: a comparison of anatomic and reverse shoulder arthroplasty. J Shoulder Elbow Surg 2015;24(6):867–74.

71. Levy JC, Everding NG, Frankle MA, et al. Accuracy of patient-specific guided glenoid baseplate positioning for reverse shoulder arthroplasty. J Shoulder Elbow Surg 2014;23(10):1563–7.

72. Throckmorton TW, Gulotta LV, Bonnarens FO, et al. Patient-specific targeting guides compared with traditional instrumentation for glenoid component placement in shoulder arthroplasty: a multi-surgeon study in 70 arthritic cadaver specimens. J Shoulder Elbow Surg 2015;24(6):965–71.

Implant Selection for Proximal Humerus Fractures

Adeshina Adeyemo, MD, BSN, Nicholas Bertha, MD, Kevin J. Perry, MD, DPT,
Gary Updegrove, MD*

KEYWORDS

- Proximal humerus fracture • Hemiarthroplasty • Locking plate • Intramedullary nail
- Reverse total shoulder arthroplasty

KEY POINTS

- Implant selection in operative proximal humerus fractures should be guided by multiple patient- and surgeon-specific factors.
- Age, physiologic status, fracture pattern, bone quality, available augments, and surgeon training should all influence decision-making.
- Multiple augments to open reduction internal fixation are available, and their indications are evolving.
- Reverse total shoulder arthroplasty is gaining traction as a reliable procedure for complex proximal humerus fractures in older patients with poor bone quality.
- Despite an abundance of evidence, the ideal treatment algorithm for proximal humerus fractures is yet to be elucidated.

INTRODUCTION

Proximal humerus fractures (PHF) are classically described based on Neer's 4-part classification, which includes the lesser tuberosity, greater tuberosity, humeral head, and humeral shaft.[1] The AO/Orthopedic Trauma Association classification defines the proximal humerus as the area within a box where the width and height are equal to the maximal width of the proximal humeral epiphysis.[2,3] PHF occur in a bimodal distribution, with one peak in young patients due to high-energy trauma and another in elderly patients with low-energy osteoporosis-related trauma. This injury occurs more often in women and incidence increases with advancing age.

Management of PHF has served as a topic of debate for years. Indications for surgery and surgical treatment options remain controversial with evidence to support many differing treatment algorithms. Dr C Michael Robinson may have said it best: "More ink than blood may have been spilt in the debate over these injuries, and their discussion in the orthopedic literature is disproportionate to their prevalence." The following review discusses the pertinent literature regarding fixation method and implant selection related to the surgical treatment of PHF. For simplicity of discussion, this review focuses on operative management alone. The authors acknowledge the evidence in support of nonoperative management of PHF and focuses on discussing implant choices once a surgical decision is made.

OPERATIVE MANAGEMENT

In general, indications for operative management of PHF may include 2-, 3-, or 4-part fractures, greater tuberosity displacement greater than 3 mm in an athlete or greater than 5 mm in adult, humeral head-split, and open fracture. Surgical options are plentiful but can be divided into 2 major categories: fracture fragment

---

Department of Bone and Joint, Penn State Milton Hershey Medical Center, 30 Hope Drive, Building A; PO Box 859, Hershey, PA 17033, USA
* Corresponding author.
E-mail address: gupdegrove@pennstatehealth.psu.edu

reduction and fixation versus arthroplasty. Reduction and fixation can be accomplished with several implants including pins, suture fixation, flexible nails, plates and screws, and locked intramedullary nails (IMNs). Arthroplasty options are typically reserved to hemiarthroplasty and reverse total shoulder arthroplasty.

Selection of treatment and implants may be attributed to patient-, injury-, and surgeon-specific factors. Patient conditions include physiologic age, functional status, and bone quality. Injury-specific factors include fracture pattern, displacement, vascularity, and rotator cuff integrity. Surgeon training, volume, and practice location may also affect implant choice.

Fixation Versus Arthroplasty

Decision-making regarding implant selection must first begin with selection of fracture fragment fixation or arthroplasty. Hertel investigated risk factors for avascular necrosis (AVN) of the humeral head based on fracture pattern.[4] In his study, drill holes were made in the humeral head at the time of fixation, and return of blood was considered intact vascular supply. Patients were followed radiographically to look for signs of AVN in order to describe predictors of ischemia. Disruption of the medial hinge, metaphyseal extension of the humeral head less than 8 mm, and complex fracture patterns were good predictors of ischemia.[5] The combination of all of the criteria had a positive predictive value of greater than 97% for developing humeral head ischemia.[5] In 2015, Campochiaro and colleagues[5] evaluated 250 PHF using Hertel's criteria that were treated by open reduction and internal fixation (ORIF). They found the rate of AVN of the humeral head to be 3.7%, with no significant correlation to fracture type or gender. They also found that in the AVN group, only 30% of the patients presented with all of Hertel's criteria. As a result, the investigators had concern in their ability to accurately identify the calcar segment and recommended for surgeons to pursue 3-dimensional computerized tomography imaging to better determine fracture pattern. Batsian and colleagues[6] showed that intraoperative assessment of vascularity via drill holes was not a reliable predictor of AVN at long-term follow-up drawing further questions to Hertel's criteria. Head-split fractures and fracture dislocations were once thought to be significant risk factors for AVN; however, modern studies show low rates of AVN with both patterns as long as the capsule remains attached to the fracture fragments.[4,7,8] Although AVN can be detrimental to outcomes, it should also not be the only predictor used in surgical decision-making. Interestingly, Gerber and colleagues[9] showed that in patients with AVN without malunion, outcomes were reasonable; however, patients with AVN and malunion had poor outcomes.

Other factors that drive decision-making include patient age, physiologic status, bone quality, and smoking status. Increased patient age is a predictor for loss of reduction, screw cut-out, and increased complications overall with ORIF.[10,11] Complications are also increased in older patients after shoulder arthroplasty.[12] In most series, patients aged 60 to 70 years and beyond portend worse outcomes with fixation compared with arthroplasty[10,13]; however, other studies suggest similar outcomes should proper ORIF techniques be used.[14] There is no definitive consensus, however, and many surgeons prefer arthroplasty for older patients. Smoking is a risk factor for nonunion with fixation.[15–17]

Osteoporosis is a risk factor for loss of reduction and malunion with fixation. Several attempts have been made to quantify bone quality in the proximal humerus including the Deltoid Tuberosity Index (DTI)[18] and combined cortical thickness (CCT).[19] DTI is calculated by measuring the outer cortical diameter and the endosteal width just proximal to the deltoid tuberosity.[18] CCT involves measuring the medial and lateral cortical thickness at 2 specific levels of the proximal humeral diaphysis. These measurements correlate to bone mineral density and can help guide treatment.[19] Decreased bone mineral density is associated with screw cut-out and loss of reduction.[20]

Attempts have been made at defining an evidence-based treatment algorithm for PHF. Spross and colleagues[18] published a prospective study in which they created an algorithm to treat patients with PHF. Considerations for their algorithm included patient's age, fracture pattern, bone quality, and functional status.[16,18] Their treatment algorithm pursued nonoperative management for 1-part fractures. For 2-part fractures in young and older patients, ORIF with augmentation was indicated. For 3- and 4-part, or head-split fractures in young patients, hemiarthroplasty (HA) was performed. In older patients with 3- and 4-part fractures, or head-split fractures, reverse total shoulder arthroplasty (RSA) was the treatment of choice. Surgeon adherence to their algorithm was 83%. Patients treated by their algorithm had a mean relative Constant score of 95% at 1 year.

To further complicate the decision-making process is the outcomes data of delayed shoulder arthroplasty. In some series, reverse shoulder arthroplasty performed for revision of fixation failure or for failed nonoperative treatment had similar outcomes to primary reverse shoulder arthroplasty. Dezfuli and colleagues compared outcomes between primary reverse for fracture versus reverse for failed ORIF and reverse for failed hemiarthroplasty. The primary reverse group had comparable outcomes to salvage for failed ORIF. The failed hemiarthroplasty group had the worst overall function following revision to reverse.[21] Therefore, when the implant choice is difficult, attempting fixation may be a reasonable strategy knowing that the patient's ultimate function can be salvaged if fixation fails.[22]

Open Reduction and Internal Fixation with Plates and Screws

ORIF is generally indicated for patients younger than 65 years with good bone stock and high physiologic demand.[23,24] Nonlocking plates have high rates of failure and lower biomechanical strength compared with locking plates and are no longer recommended in the treatment of PHF.[25] Locking plates have a high rate of reoperation (16%–30%) largely due to screw cut-out and plate impingement.[26]

Generally, ORIF with plates and screws is recommended for young patients with good bone quality; however there is literature advocating that locking fixed-angle plating systems may have satisfactory outcomes in elderly populations. Gavaskar and colleagues[27] followed elderly patients (older than 70 years and active) with displaced 3- and 4-part PHF treated with a second-generation proximal humerus locked plating. Results of their study revealed fracture union in 24 of 26 patients.

For younger patients with a head-split fractures pattern, ORIF remains a viable option. Gavaskar and colleagues[27] followed a series of head-split fractures and found satisfactory outcomes with ORIF for simple head-split patterns.[28] However, complex head-split fracture patterns demonstrated higher rates of AVN and worse shoulder functional outcomes.[27,28]

Several aspects of the surgical technique for open reduction and internal locking plate fixation have been linked to outcomes. Achieving anatomic reduction is important, particularly at the medial metaphysis. Lee and Shin evaluated prognostic factors for unstable PHF treated by locking plate and found that restoring the medial metaphysis was a reliable indicator of successful patient outcomes.[29] Screws should be appropriately seated in the plate while avoiding cross-threading, as this is associated with increased rate of varus collapse.[30] Another critical aspect of screw placement is the medial column screw.[27,28] The medial column screw should be placed as close to the calcar as possible and not above it to prevent the loss of reduction and collapse.[25,28–30] Variable angle screws inserted off-axis are biomechanically less stable than nominally placed screws.[30] Therefore, plate positioning should be optimized so that screws can be placed at their nominal angulation and still capture the medial calcar.

Augmentation to Open Reduction and Internal Fixation

There are various supplemental fixation methods that can be used in conjunction with ORIF. The most common techniques include suture augmentation, cement augmentation, fibular strut allografts, and nitinol cage implants. In general, augmentation is used for comminuted fractures with disruption of the medial calcar. The purpose of augmentation is to provide additional structural support to prevent collapse and loss of reduction due to the collapse of the osteopenic humeral head and metaphyseal bone.

Tension band suture fixation has been shown to improve union rates by aiding in countering the deforming forces of the rotator cuff muscle on the tuberosity fragments.[31] In theory, suture fixation also provides additional stabilization strength without having to rely entirely on screw purchase in osteoporotic bone. Shukla and colleagues performed suture augmentation of the rotator cuff (RTC) for 2-, 3-, and 4-part PHF. Their study results suggested that suture augmentation of the RTC counteracts varus forces on PHF stabilized by locking plates and should be routinely performed in 2-, 3-, and 4-part fractures.[32]

The use of a fibular strut allograft remains controversial, although may be helpful in patients with poor bone quality and in fracture patterns in which the medial metaphysis cannot be anatomically reduced. This involves placement of a short segment of fibula with 2 to 3 cm of graft proximal to the surgical neck. The graft is used to help reduce and support the calcar.[33,34] This technique can be beneficial in comminuted PHF and help maintain anatomic reduction and reduce the change in humeral height.[35–37] A systematic review by Saltzman and colleagues[35] looked into 4 fibular strut studies and showed the rate of screw penetration was 3.7% and the rate of reoperation was 4.4%. These rates were much lower than rates seen in prior studies with typical plating techniques. One concern in regard to the use of fibular strut allografts is their incorporation into the intramedullary canal. In the event of revision to arthroplasty, the fibula graft can be exceedingly difficult to remove from the canal, which may be necessary to appropriately place the humeral component.

Cement augmentation is another method used to minimize fracture settling and screw cut-out in the setting of poor bone quality. Calcium phosphate or polymethylmethacrylate (PMMA) can be injected along the screw tracts before screw insertion as augmentation. Egol and colleagues[38] showed a significant decrease in screw cut-out with cement augmentation of PHF treated with locked plate fixation.

Cage implants are a more recently described technique for medial calcar support in complex PHF. The indications are not yet clear, but this technique is most commonly used for PHF with a varus deformity, calcar comminution, 3- and 4-part fractures, and also osteoporotic bone. In comparison to traditional ORIF, cage implants have been shown to have lower rates of reoperation at the first year, according to the case series by Goodnough and colleagues.[39] Hudgens and colleagues[40] followed-up 11 patients with either a 3- or a 4-part fracture that was treated with cage augmentation and found successful patient outcomes (American shoulder and elbow surgeons score; subjective shoulder value) and 100% union rate. However, similar to fibular strut allograft, their use in fracture fixation can make later revision to arthroplasty difficult.

Intramedullary Nail

IMNs continue to be used by some surgeons for proximal humerus fracture fixation, both with closed as well open reduction techniques. IMN is most commonly used for 2-part fractures usually located at the surgical neck. However, IMN may be used for more complex fractures with the addition of proximal poly angle locking screws for tuberosity fixation.[25] One advantage of an IMN is that it provides more stability and stiffness compared with plate fixation or pinning.[41] Newer IMN designs have minimized rotator cuff morbidity and iatrogenic fractures by reducing exposure requirements and changing nail designs to allow for a more medial insertion through the musculature of the supraspinatus in order to avoid insertion through the rotator cuff tendon footprint.[42] Outcomes for IMN have been shown to have no difference when compared with ORIF with plates and screws,[24] and some studies have even shown that there is a reduced rate of complications compared with ORIF.[43] Yiming and colleagues

conducted a prospective randomized controlled trial in which they compared outcomes for treatment of 2-part PHF using locked IMN versus locking plates. There was not a statistically significant difference between both groups in active range of motion 3 years after the procedure.[43] In the same study, the strength of the supraspinatus in the IMN group was less than that of the locked plate group, although this was also not statistically significant. The investigators concluded that IMNs are most beneficial when used for 2-part surgical neck fractures with an intact osseous ring.[43]

Traditionally, the insertion point of humeral nails was through the supraspinatus tendon at the footprint on the greater tuberosity; however, newer generations of nails now use a more medial starting point. The medial starting point is at the lateral edge of the humeral head articular surface. The purpose of this entry point is to attempt to avoid the supraspinatus tendon by allowing passage of the nail through the muscle fibers in an effort to minimize long-term pain from supraspinatus tendinopathy and tears.[25]

Gadea and colleagues examined radiologic markers comparing plate fixation versus IMN and found that fractures with an intact medial hinge had better functional outcomes when fixed with locking plate and screws. Otherwise ORIF and IMN has similar anatomic reduction rates and functional outcomes.[44]

Percutaneous Fixation

Percutaneous pinning is another option for treatment of PHF and results in a construct to provide stability but does not provide a significant amount of stiffness.[45] One of the benefits of percutaneous pinning is that it offers a minimally invasive option for stabilization. Percutaneous pinning is most often performed in patients with good bone stock, an intact medial calcar, and typically for 2-part fractures.[46] Outcomes have not been shown to be as successful for patients with 3-part fractures.[47] Percutaneous fixation is technically challenging with difficulties obtaining and maintaining an appropriate reduction. Axillary and radial nerve palsies have been described following this procedure.[48]

Another minimally invasive option is flexible IMNs, sometimes referred to as Zifko nails. The flexible nails are inserted retrograde through the intramedullary canal, and a bouquet of multiple nails is affected into the humeral head once a closed or percutaneous reduction is achieved. A study by Matziolis and colleagues[49] using Zifko nails has shown clinical outcomes and complication rates similar to fixed angle plating.

External Fixation

The external fixator is rarely used in the modern surgical treatment of PHF. It provides limited stability comparable to percutaneous pins. The benefit of the external fixator is that it is applied percutaneously and allows for early mobilization. External fixation has similar limitations to percutaneous pin fixation. Parlato and colleagues[50] describe a series of 84 patients treated with external fixation with successful outcomes in 2- and 3-part fractures. External fixation is not routinely used in the management of PHF; however, it remains an option in a wide array of PHF fixation strategies.

Arthroplasty

Shoulder arthroplasty has become a common treatment of PHF as well as proximal humerus fracture sequelae. Relative indications for arthroplasty include 3- or 4-part fractures, head-split fractures, and fracture dislocations. Its use is typically reserved for older patients with lower functional demands. According to Krishnan and colleagues,[51] patients older than 70 years should undergo arthroplasty rather than ORIF due to their poor neuromuscular control and poor bone quality. Arthroplasty options in the setting of fracture are often reserved to HA or RSA. Despite arthroplasty becoming more commonly used in the setting of acute PHF, some studies suggest that joint preserving treatments yield higher postsurgical Constant scores.[52,53]

In young patients with severely comminuted humeral head fragments, hemiarthroplasty is a surgical treatment option. However, functional outcome heavily depends on anatomic reduction and healing of the tuberosities.[34] Tuberosity malunion has been shown to be a source of failure following HA.[54] A retrospective study by Boileau and colleagues[54] showed that 42% of

Table 1
Pros and cons of operative management options for proximal humerus fractures

Fixation Method	Pros	Cons
Closed reduction percutaneous pinning	• Minimally invasive • Good stability	• Higher failure rates in 3-part fractures • Limited stiffness • Technically challenging for maintaining reduction • Higher risks of nerve palsies
Zipfko nails	• Minimally invasive	• Limited indications • Low stiffness
External fixation	• Minimally invasive • Allows early mobilization	• Low stability • Limited indications
Locking plate ± suture augmentation	• Highly versatile based on fracture pattern	• Requires good bone stock
Locking plate + intramedullary fibular graft	• Provides medial calcar support	• Challenging revision
Locking plate + intramedullary cage	• Provides medial calcar support	• Challenging revision
Locking plate + PMMA cement augment	• Provides medial calcar support • Decreased screw cut-out	• Challenging revision
Intramedullary locking nail	• Increased stability and stiffness • May have reduced complications compared with ORIF	• Rotator cuff morbidity
Hemiarthroplasty	• Useful for comminuted fractures	• High failure rates in elderly • Requires an intact rotator cuff
Reverse shoulder arthroplasty	• Good for improving pain • Can be used if patient has a concurrent rotator cuff tear • Provides a viable salvage procedure	• Patient needs to be able to tolerate restrictions • Specific complications related to RSA

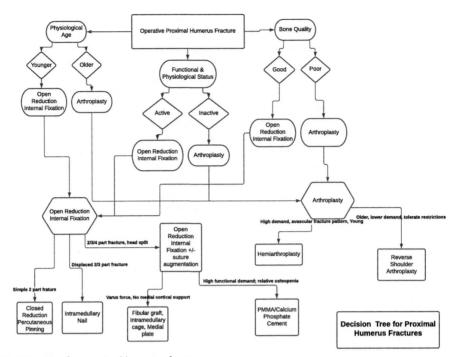

Fig. 1. Decision tree for proximal humerus fractures.

patients who underwent HA were not satisfied with the surgical outcome. The incidence of tuberosity malposition was up to 50%. HA is not typically chosen as a first option, and there are studies showing that HA provides no clear benefit over nonoperative management, when the patient is older than 65 years.[55] HA is primarily reserved for young patients with high functional demand in the setting of a proximal humerus fracture that cannot be anatomically reconstructed and stabilized by ORIF.

Older patients with PHF and poor bone quality may be treated surgically with reverse total shoulder arthroplasty. Reverse shoulder arthroplasty has been shown to have reliable results, which makes it an enticing option for PHF management.[56] Functional outcomes of reverse shoulder arthroplasty are less dependent on tuberosity positioning and healing than hemiarthroplasty.[57] Attempts should still be made to reduce and repair the tuberosities, as several series have shown improved outcomes with RSA with healed tuberosities.[57–59] It is imperative to evaluate the patient for an axillary nerve palsy before RSA and to ensure appropriate deltoid function, which is essential for successful outcome with reverse shoulder arthroplasty.[60]

A systematic review by Mata-Fink and colleagues[61] showed that RSA had superior outcomes to HA. There is mixed evidence regarding timing of RSA and outcomes, but in general, studies have not shown significant differences between reverse for acute fracture versus reverse for failed ORIF.[21] Some studies suggest increased range of motion and tuberosity union rate when performed acutely.[62,63] Overall, there seems to be reasonable outcomes for RSA when performed both primarily and secondarily as a salvage procedure after failure of fixation.[64]

Compared with reverse for cuff tear arthropathy, reverse for fracture has a higher complication rate. Patients typically have an increased risk of transfusion, longer length of stay, and are more likely to be discharged to extended care facilities.[65] Interestingly, these data seem to mirror trends seen in hip arthroplasty literature comparing elective total hip arthroplasty for osteoarthritis with acute total hip arthroplasty for femoral neck fractures.

SUMMARY

Unfortunately, there is not enough clear evidence to support a specific treatment algorithm for the surgical management of PHF at this time. Despite evidence to suggest vascularity may be preserved in fracture patterns including Hertel's criteria, head-split fractures, and fracture dislocations, these patterns are perceived to support the use of arthroplasty. Future research is necessary to delineate more specific risk factors for

AVN and fixation failure. Further clarification is necessary regarding outcomes of RSA for failed fixation versus primary reverse for fracture, as this may help to shape future decision-making. To help illustrate the fine points discussed in this article, **Table 1** and **Fig. 1** discuss fixation methods and their pros and cons and also a decision tree to follow, in regard to how to operatively manage PHF.

Despite extensive research on the topic of implant selection for management of PHF, there remains no single optimal surgical treatment algorithm. Evidence supports the use of multiple patient-, injury-, and surgeon-related factors in surgical decision-making. These include age, physiologic status, fracture pattern, bone quality, and surgeon experience. Although the optimal management of PHF remains unclear, good patient outcomes can be achieved through a variety of techniques.

CLINICS CARE POINTS

- Operative management of PHF should be tailored to patient-specific factors (age, functional status, fracture pattern, and bone quality).

- An evidence-based algorithmic approach to PHF may optimize outcomes.

DISCLOSURE

G. Updegrove: Consultant for Aevumed.

REFERENCES

1. Carofino BC, Leopold SS. 2013. Classifications in brief: the Neer classification for proximal humerus fractures. Clin Orthop Relat Res 2013;471(1):39–43.

2. Meinberg EG, Agel J, Roberts CS, et al. Fracture and dislocation classification compendium-2018. J Orthop Trauma 2018;32(Suppl 1):S1–170.

3. AO Foundation. AO/OTA fracture and dislocation classification: introduction to the classification of long-bone fractures. Switzerland; 2020. Available at: https://www2.aofoundation.org/AOFileServer-Surgery/MyPortalFiles?FilePath=/Surgery/en/_docs/AOOTA%20Classification%20Compendium%202018.pdf. Accessed November 10, 2020.

4. Hertel R, Hempfing A, Stiehler M, et al. Predictors of humeral head ischemia after intracapsular fracture of the proximal humerus. J Shoulder Elbow Surg 2004;13(4):427–33.

5. Campochiaro G, Rebuzzi M, Baudi P, et al. Complex proximal humerus fractures: Hertel's criteria reliability to predict head necrosis. Musculoskelet Surg 2015;99(Suppl 1):S9–15.

6. Bastian JD, Hertel R. Initial post-fracture humeral head ischemia does not predict development of necrosis. J Shoulder Elbow Surg 2008;17(1):2–8.

7. Robinson CM, Khan LA, Akhtar MA. Treatment of anterior fracture-dislocations of the proximal humerus by open reduction and internal fixation. J Bone Joint Surg Br 2006;88(4):502–8.

8. Large TM, Adams MR, Loeffler BJ, et al. Posttraumatic avascular necrosis after proximal femur, proximal humerus, talar neck, and scaphoid fractures. J Am Acad Orthop Surg 2019;27(21):794–805.

9. Gerber C, Hersche O, Berberat C. The clinical relevance of posttraumatic avascular necrosis of the humeral head. J Shoulder Elbow Surg 1998;7(6):586–90.

10. Klug A, Wincheringer D, Harth J, et al. Complications after surgical treatment of proximal humerus fractures in the elderly—an analysis of complication patterns and risk factors for reverse shoulder arthroplasty and angular-stable plating. J Shoulder Elbow Surg 2019;28(9):1674–84.

11. Jost B, Spross C, Grehn H, et al. Locking plate fixation of fractures of the proximal humerus: analysis of complications, revision strategies and outcome. J Shoulder Elbow Surg 2013;22(4):542–9.

12. Wall B, Walch G. Reverse shoulder arthroplasty for the treatment of proximal humeral fractures. Hand Clin 2007;23(4):425–30.

13. Du S, Ye J, Chen H, et al. Interventions for Treating 3-or 4-part proximal humeral fractures in elderly patient: a network meta-analysis of randomized controlled trials. Int J Surg 2017;48:240–6.

14. Schliemann B, Siemoneit J, Theisen C, et al. Complex fractures of the proximal humerus in the elderly—outcome and complications after locking plate fixation. Musculoskelet Surg 2012;96(1):3–11.

15. Boesmueller S, Wech M, Gregori M, et al. Risk factors for humeral head necrosis and non-union after plating in proximal humeral fractures. Injury 2016;47(2):350–5.

16. Rose PS, Adams CR, Torchia ME, et al. Locking plate fixation for proximal humeral fractures: initial results with a new implant. J Shoulder Elbow Surg 2007;16(2):202–7.

17. Spross C, Platz A, Rufibach K, et al. The PHILOS plate for proximal humeral fractures—risk factors for complications at one year. J Trauma Acute Care Surg 2012;72(3):783–92.

18. Spross C, Kaestle N, Benninger E, et al. Deltoid tuberosity index: a simple radiographic tool to assess local bone quality in proximal humerus fractures. Clin Orthop Relat Res 2015;473(9):3038–45.

19. Tingart MJ, Apreleva M, von Stechow D, et al. The cortical thickness of the proximal humeral diaphysis predicts bone mineral density of the proximal humerus. J Bone Joint Surg Br 2003;85(4):611–7.

20. Spross C, Zeledon R, Zdravkovic V, et al. How bone quality may influence intraoperative and early post-operative problems after angular stable open reduction-internal fixation of proximal humeral fractures. J Shoulder Elbow Surg 2017;26(9):1566–72.

21. Dezfuli B, King JJ, Farmer KW, et al. Outcomes of reverse total shoulder arthroplasty as primary versus revision procedure for proximal humerus fractures. J Shoulder Elbow Surg 2016;25(7):1133–7.

22. Shannon SF, Wagner ER, Houdek MT, et al. Reverse shoulder arthroplasty for proximal humeral fractures: outcomes comparing primary reverse arthroplasty for fracture versus reverse arthroplasty after failed osteosynthesis. J Shoulder Elbow Surg 2016;25(10):1655–60.

23. Choi S, Kang H, Bang H. Technical tips: dualplate fixation technique for comminuted proximal humerus fractures. Injury 2014;45(8):1280–2.

24. Dietz SO, Hartmann F, Schwarz T, et al. Retrograde nailing versus locking plate osteosynthesis of proximal humeral fractures: a biomechanical study. J Shoulder Elbow Surg 2012;21(5):618–24.

25. Dilisio MF, Nowinski RJ, Hatzidakis AM, et al. Intramedullary nailing of the proximal humerus: evolution, technique, and results. J Shoulder Elbow Surg 2016;25(5):e130–8.

26. Owsley KC, Gorczyca JT. Displacement/screw cutout after open reduction and locked plate fixation of humeral fractures. J Bone Joint Surg Am 2008;90(2):233–40.

27. Gavaskar AS, Tummala NC, Srinivasan P, et al. Second generation locked plating for complex proximal humerus fractures in very elderly patients. Injury 2016;47(11):2534–8.

28. Gavaskar AS, Tummala NC. Locked plate osteosynthesis of humeral head–splitting fractures in young adults. J Shoulder Elbow Surg 2015;24(6):908–14.

29. Lee CW, Shin SJ. Prognostic factors for unstable proximal humeral fractures treated with locking-plate fixation. J Shoulder Elbow Surg 2009;18(1):83–8.

30. Fletcher JW, Windolf M, Richards RG, et al. Screw configuration in proximal humerus plating has a significant impact on fixation failure risk predicted by finite element models. J Shoulder Elbow Surg 2019;28(9):1816–23.

31. Badman B, Frankle M, Keating C, et al. Results of proximal humeral locked plating with supplemental suture fixation of rotator cuff. J Shoulder Elbow Surg 2011;20(4):616–24.

32. Shukla DR, McAnany S, Pean C, et al. The results of tension band rotator cuff suture fixation of locked plating of displaced proximal humerus fractures. Injury 2017;48(2):474–80.

33. Bae JH, Oh JK, Chon CS, et al. The biomechanical performance of locking plate fixation with intramedullary fibular strut graft augmentation in the treatment of unstable fractures of the proximal humerus. J Bone Joint Surg Br 2011;93(7):937–41.

34. Schumaier A, Grawe B. Proximal humerus fractures: evaluation and management in the elderly patient. Geriatr Orthop Surg Rehabil 2018;9. 2151458517750516.

35. Saltzman BM, Erickson BJ, Harris JD, et al. Fibular strut graft augmentation for open reduction and internal fixation of proximal humerus fractures: a systematic review and the authors' preferred surgical technique. Orthop J Sports Med 2016;4(7). 2325967116656829.

36. Gardner MJ, Boraiah S, Helfet DL, et al. Indirect medial reduction and strut support of proximal humerus fractures using an endosteal implant. J Orthop Trauma 2008;22(3):195–200.

37. Matassi F, Angeloni R, Carulli C, et al. Locking plate and fibular allograft augmentation in unstable fractures of proximal humerus. Injury 2012;43(11):1939–42.

38. Egol KA, Sugi MT, Ong CC, et al. Fracture site augmentation with calcium phosphate cement reduces screw penetration after open reduction-internal fixation of proximal humeral fractures. J Shoulder Elbow Surg 2012;21(6):741–8.

39. Goodnough LH, Campbell ST, Githens TC, et al. Intramedullary cage fixation for proximal humerus fractures has low reoperation rates at 1 year: results of a multicenter study. J Orthop Trauma 2020;34(4):193–8.

40. Hudgens JL, Jang J, Aziz K, et al. Three-and 4-part proximal humeral fracture fixation with an intramedullary cage: 1-year clinical and radiographic outcomes. J Shoulder Elbow Surg 2019;28(6):S131–7.

41. Yoon RS, Dziadosz D, Porter DA, et al. A comprehensive update on current fixation options for two-part proximal humerus fractures: a biomechanical investigation. Injury 2014;45(3):510–4.

42. Sobel AD, Shah KN, Paxton ES. Fixation of a proximal humerus fracture with an intramedullary nail. J Orthop Trauma 2017;31(Suppl 3):S47–9.

43. Zhu Y, Lu Y, Shen J, et al. Locking intramedullary nails and locking plates in the treatment of two-part proximal humeral surgical neck fractures. J Bone Joint Surg Am 2011;93:159–68.

44. Gadea F, Favard L, Boileau P, et al. Fixation of 4-part fractures of the proximal humerus: can we identify radiological criteria that support locking plates or IM nailing? Comparative, retrospective study of 107 cases. Orthop Traumatol Surg Res 2016;102(8):963–70.

45. Lill H, Hepp P, Korner J, et al. Proximal humeral fractures: how stiff should an implant be? Arch Orthop Trauma Surg 2003;123(2–3):74–81.

46. Omid R, Galatz LM. Percutaneous pinning of proximal humerus fractures: a technique. Semin Arthroplasty 2011;22(No. 1):2–4. WB Saunders.

47. Fenichel I, Oran A, Burstein G, et al. Percutaneous pinning using threaded pins as a treatment option for unstable two-and three-part fractures of the proximal humerus: a retrospective study. Int Orthop 2006;30(3):153–7.

48. Fink Barnes L, Parsons BO, Flatow EL. Percutaneous fixation of proximal humeral fractures. JBJS Essent Surg Tech 2015;5(2):e10.

49. Matziolis D, Kaeaeb M, Zandi SS, et al. Surgical treatment of two-part fractures of the proximal humerus: comparison of fixed-angle plate osteosynthesis and Zifko nails. Injury 2010;41(10):1041–6.

50. Parlato A, D'Arienzo A, Ferruzza M, et al. Indications and limitations of the fixator TGF "Gex-Fix" in proximal end humeral fractures. Injury 2014;45: S49–52.

51. Krishnan SG, Bennion PW, Reineck JR, et al. Hemiarthroplasty for proximal humeral fracture: restoration of the Gothic arch. Orthop Clin North Am 2008;39(4):441–50, vi.

52. Gomberawalla MM, Miller BS, Coale RM, et al. Meta-analysis of joint preservation versus arthroplasty for the treatment of displaced 3-and 4-part fractures of the proximal humerus. Injury 2013; 44(11):1532–9.

53. den Hartog D, de Haan J, Schep NW, et al. Primary shoulder arthroplasty versus conservative treatment for comminuted proximal humeral fractures: a systematic literature review. Open Orthop J 2010;4:87.

54. Boileau P, Krishnan SG, Tinsi L, et al. Tuberosity malposition and migration: Reasons for poor outcomes 48. after hemiarthroplasty for displaced fractures of the proximal humerus. J Shoulder Elbow Surg 2002;11(5):401–12.

55. Olerud P, Ahrengart L, Ponzer S, et al. Hemiarthroplasty versus nonoperative treatment of displaced 4-part proximal humeral fractures in elderly patients: a randomized controlled trial. J Shoulder Elbow Surg 2011;20(7):1025–33.

56. Sershon RA, Van Thiel GS, Lin EC, et al. Clinical outcomes of reverse total shoulder arthroplasty in patients aged younger than 60 years. J Shoulder Elbow Surg 2014;23(3):395–400.

57. Boileau P, Alta TD, Decroocq L, et al. Reverse shoulder arthroplasty for acute fractures in the elderly: is it worth reattaching the tuberosities? J Shoulder Elbow Surg 2019;28(3):437–44.

58. Ohl X, Bonnevialle N, Gallinet D, et al. How the greater tuberosity affects clinical outcomes after reverse shoulder arthroplasty for proximal humeral fractures. J Shoulder Elbow Surg 2018;27(12):2139–44.

59. Barros LH, Figueiredo S, Marques M, et al. Tuberosity healinh after reverse shoulder arthroplasty for proximal humerus Fractures: Is there clinical improvement? Rev Bras Ortop. 2019 Aug 15. Available at: https://www.thieme-connect.de/products/ejournals/pdf/10.1055/s-0039-3402459.pdf?articleLanguage=en. Accessed November 10, 2020.

60. Chae J, Siljander M, Wiater JM. Instability in reverse total shoulder arthroplasty. J Am Acad Orthop Surg 2018;26(17):587–96.

61. Mata-Fink A, Meinke M, Jones C, et al. Reverse shoulder arthroplasty for treatment of proximal humeral fractures in older adults: a systematic review. J Shoulder Elbow Surg 2013;22(12):1737–48.

62. Linkous N, Wright JO, Koueiter DM, et al. Outcomes for reverse total shoulder arthroplasty after failed open reduction internal fixation versus primary reverse total shoulder arthroplasty for proximal humerus fractures. Semin Arthroplasty 2020; 30(No. 2):111–6. WB Saunders.

63. Seidl A, Sholder D, Warrender W, et al. Early versus late reverse shoulder arthroplasty for proximal humerus fractures: does it matter? Arch Bone Jt Surg 2017;5(4):213.

64. Nelson PA, Kwan CC, Tjong VK, et al. primary versus salvage reverse total shoulder arthroplasty for displaced proximal humerus fractures in the elderly: a systematic review and Meta-analysis. Journal of shoulder and elbow arthroplasty. 2020 Sep 15. Available at: https://journals.sagepub.com/doi/10.1177/2471549220949731. Accessed November 10, 2020.

65. Liu JN, Agarwalla A, Gowd AK, et al. Reverse shoulder arthroplasty for proximal humerus fracture: a more complex episode of care than for cuff tear arthropathy. J Shoulder Elbow Surg 2019;28(11):2139–46.

Foot and Ankle

Orthopedic Versus Podiatric Care of the Foot and Ankle: A Literature Review

Charlotte Allen, MBChB, FRACS[a],
Alastair Younger, MBChB, MSc, ChM, FRCSC[b],*,
Andrea Veljkovic, MD, MPH, BComm, FRCSC[c],
Mark Glazebrook, MD, MSc, PhD, Dip Sports Med, FRCSC[d]

KEYWORDS

- Podiatry • Orthopedic • Foot and ankle surgery • Fusion • Replacement • Ankle fracture
- Pilon fracture

KEY POINTS

- Podiatric surgeons are increasing their scope of practice, and patients are more likely to be satisfied with their podiatrist than their orthopedic surgeon.
- Podiatrists are more likely to offer surgery than orthopedic surgeons.
- Per episode of care, the podiatric costs were lower; however, because multiple procedures were used to treat a single condition, the overall cost of care was higher.
- For ankle fusion podiatrists were more likely to have a complication. For ankle fractures, podiatrists are more likely to have a malunion or nonunion.
- The causes of litigation was different between podiatry and orthopedic surgery.

INTRODUCTION

Foot and ankle surgery is performed by both orthopedic surgeons and podiatrists with a significant overlap of the services provided. The training, education, and certification is different for these providers, with orthopedic surgeons training for minimum of 9 years, including medical school, and podiatrists training for 4 to 6 years, focusing on the foot and ankle only.[1] Podiatrists also have different certification requirements compared with orthopedic surgeons. It can be difficult to compare the 2 professions because, although there is overlap in procedures provided, the patient groups can vary significantly. Overall, orthopedic surgeons perform a higher volume of trauma care,[2,3] including a higher volume of surgery around the ankle, whereas podiatrists perform more toe surgery.[3,4] Because of this factor, the outcomes on a procedure basis are difficult to compare. The value proposition increasingly adopted within health care systems to achieve cost containment while improving patient outcomes places increasing pressure on foot and ankle surgical services, even as demand for services continue to grow.[3]

There are a handful of studies in the literature that attempt to identify and assess the differences between the 2 groups and compare the outcomes. The aim of this study was to systematically review the findings of these studies.

---

[a] Footbridge Clinic, Providence Healthcare, University of British Columbia, 221 - 181 Keefer Place, Vancouver, British Columbia V6B 6C1, Canada; [b] Footbridge Clinic, St Pauls Hospital, Providence Healthcare, University of British Columbia, 221 - 181 Keefer Place, Vancouver, British Columbia V6B 6C1, Canada; [c] Department of Orthopaedics, Footbridge Clinic, St Pauls Hospital, Providence Healthcare, University of British Columbia, 221 - 181 Keefer Place, Vancouver, British Columbia V6B 6C1, Canada; [d] Dalhouse University, Queen Elizabeth II Hospital, 1796 Summer Street, Halifax, Nova Scotia, B3H 3A7, Canada
* Corresponding author.
E-mail address: asyounger@shaw.ca

Orthop Clin N Am 52 (2021) 177–180
https://doi.org/10.1016/j.ocl.2020.12.004
0030-5898/21/© 2020 Elsevier Inc. All rights reserved.

METHODS

In September 2020 we searched Embase and Ovid Medline as well as bibliographies of relevant articles for comparative studies of orthopedic foot and ankle surgery and podiatry. Three of the authors (CA, AL, AV) assessed the abstracts of the articles found as well as the full text of the articles that were deemed appropriate. We included all studies that compared the aspects of orthopedic surgery in the foot and ankle with podiatry. Articles were excluded if they did not relate to surgical podiatrists.

RESULTS

The search identified 35 articles via Ovid and 87 via Embase. After removing duplicates and articles not related to the research question, 13 articles were reviewed in full and 10 of these were included in this systematic review. The selected studies were written between 1987 and 2020, originating from the United States and the United Kingdom (Table 1). The clinical roles of podiatrists and orthopedic surgeons in the United States and UK were felt to be similar enough to allow a pooled analysis of these data.

Volumes and Scope of Practice and Surgery Type

Podiatrists have been shown to recommend surgery more often than orthopedic surgeons for a given patient demographic. When a second opinion was performed by an orthopedic surgeon on a case indicated by a podiatrist, a significant decrease in the number of cases indicated for surgery resulted. Podiatrists confirmed surgery in 94.3% of cases compared with 49.5% of the cases seen by orthopedic surgeons[5] Orthopedic surgeons are more likely to operate on acute cases than podiatrists,[2,3] with 1 study showing that 94.3% of the total cases performed by podiatrists were for hallux valgus, whereas orthopedic surgeons' most common procedure was for ankle fractures.[3]

Podiatrists Have Had Increasing Involvement in the Hospital Care of Patients

Surgical volume for both groups is gradually increasing, with a reported 82% increase in ankle fracture surgeries between 2005 and 2015.[3,6,7] This number reflects an increase of 424% for podiatrists and 72% for orthopedic surgeons. Pilon fracture fixation over the same time period increased by 386% for podiatrists and 103% for orthopedic surgeons.[3] In another study, ankle fracture fixation by podiatrists increased from 3.5% to 7.0% between 2007 and 2015.[6]

Over a 5-year period at a level I trauma center, the podiatry share of consultations increased from 9% to 58% of all consultations.[7] Podiatry was only in the hospital during daytime hours and, therefore, their referrals only occurred between 8 AM and 6 PM. The majority of surgical cases were managed by orthopedic surgeons; however, this proportion decreased from 92% to 59% over the 5*year period as podiatrists took on more cases.[7] Podiatrists are also starting to perform more specialized procedures such as total ankle replacements (TAA), with 1 study showing an increase from 12.8% to 24.6% of annual TAA volume and 13.6% to 26.0% of ankle arthrodesis volume over 5 years. In this study, podiatrists tended to treat more obese patients and those who were on average sicker.[8]

Podiatrists were more likely to operate on the lesser toes[4] and orthopedic surgeons were more likely to operate on other parts of the foot.

Factors identified with an increased probability of a patient having surgery by a podiatrist were older age, in areas of higher podiatrist and lower orthopedic surgeon to population ratio, and in states with more permissive regulations for podiatric surgery.[9]

Cost

Podiatrists were more likely to order additional tests than orthopedic surgeons, which would have additional costs associated.[5] They were also shown to accept lower reimbursement rates from insurance providers, billing on average $2700 and accepting an average payment of $1169.[5]

For podiatrists, compared with orthopedic surgeons performing ankle arthrodesis and total ankle arthroplasty, patients had a longer length of stay (14% longer), readmission rates, and higher cost of hospitalization for total ankle arthroplasty (28% higher at $19,236 vs $13,433) as well as a nonsignificant increased opioid utilization (+10.9%)[8]

Orthopedic surgeons compared with podiatrists in 1987 were more likely to use the inpatient setting ranging from 5.6 times (soft tissue) and 2.5 times (bunions). Orthopedic surgeons' patients also had a longer length of stay for each procedure. Podiatrists were more likely to perform a greater number of procedures per episode and perform more than 1 day of surgery per patient. The per-procedure charges were similar between the 2 groups but overall the podiatrist's episodes were more expensive owing to the multiple procedures and the involvement of assistant surgeons more commonly.[9]

Cost differences were further described in another study. Podiatrists had a lower charge per procedure (12%) but an increased charge per episode of care ($665 vs $466). They performed more procedures per episode (5.9 vs 3.9). There were similar average adjusted length of stays between the 2 groups.[10]

Outcomes

Foot and ankle surgery has significant variation in outcomes and litigation is common, because consenting can be difficult. In a study by Hartnett and associates,[2] malpractice litigation was assessed between 2004 and 2017. Podiatrists were found to be involved in 76.4% of the cases.[2] The most common cause for litigation in both groups was pain. The second most common cause for litigation was surgical complications in the surgeon group and deformity in the podiatry group. The top plaintiff allegations were failure to treat the patient (45.5%) and inappropriate surgical procedure for podiatrists. For orthopedic surgeons, the most common allegations were improper surgical procedure, intraoperative error and improper postsurgical care at 27.3% each.[2] There were no significant differences reported in case outcomes between the specialties. Trauma care in general has higher litigation rates, and because podiatry has less involvement in this area of practice, litigation rates may not be comparable.

Chan and colleagues[6] compared podiatrists' and orthopedic surgeons' complication rates after ankle fixation. Malunion or nonunion was found to be significantly higher in the fractures operated on by podiatrists compared with orthopedic surgeons with a relative risk of 1.6 when treated by podiatrists. Comparing bimalleolar and trimalleolar fractures, the relative risk of malunion/nonunion increases to 1.7 when treated by podiatrists compared with orthopedic surgeons. No significant differences were found in other postoperative complications.[6]

In comparing podiatrists and orthopedic surgeons performing ankle arthrodesis and TAA, an increased length of stay and cost of hospitalization was associated with cases performed by the podiatrists[8]

Laxton and colleagues[4] showed an 86% patient satisfaction rate with podiatrists and a 69% rate for other surgeons (orthopedic and general) when performing operations of the feet, with complaints mostly relating to lack of postoperative assistance and follow-up.

DISCUSSION

Orthopedic surgery and podiatry have significant overlap in services provided. This situation is unusual because of the significantly different training pathways. Undergraduate training is relatively similar in terms of basic science curriculum, except that podiatry concentrates on the foot and ankle. Residency training differs significantly.[1] In the United States, certification for orthopedic surgeons is by the Medical Board of Medical Specialties. With the variation in studies within this review, it is not known if the orthopedic surgeons are all specifically foot and ankle fellowship trained. Podiatrist can be certified by 2 boards in 3 specialty areas.

In a number of states, podiatrists are not allowed to operate under general anesthetic, so procedures are performed under local anesthetic blocks.

The patient groups managed by podiatrists and orthopedic surgeons are significantly different. More forefoot and toe surgery is performed by podiatrists, whereas more trauma and ankle surgeries are performed by orthopedic surgeons.[2–4] These differences make a comparison of the groups difficult.

The demand for foot and ankle surgery is increasing and putting pressure on already stretched resources.[3] Podiatrists have been able to help with the load by increasing their scope of practice to include more ankle fractures as well as ankle fusion and TAA.[3,6,7]

Cost containment is also an important issue in the current climate. Costs are relatively difficult to compare between the 2 groups because of the different patient populations served and surgical procedures performed.

For fear of litigation, many investigators are reluctant to publish on the outcomes comparing

Table 1 Details of included studies	
Study	**Country**
Laughlin et al,[1] 1996	United States
Hartnett et al,[2] 2020	United States
Burton et al,[3] 2020	United States
Laxton et al,[4] 1995	UK
Chan et al,[6] 2019	United States
Harris et al,[10] 1997	United States
Wiener 1987	United States
Jakoi et al,[7] 2014	United States
Finkel et al,[5] 1982	United States
Chan et al,[8] 2019	United States

the 2 surgeon types. However, this research is as important as any other outcomes research because both providers and patients alike need to be informed of the manageable risk factors in the provision of care.

SUMMARY

Podiatrists have an expanding scope of practice in foot and ankle surgery with increasing overlap with orthopedic surgeons. Patients are more satisfied with the care of podiatrists however overall costs of care are higher. There are increased complications following surgery by podiatrists in more complex cases.

CLINICS CARE POINTS

- To reduce litigation, surgeons should consider improving pre-operative education on expectations following surgery particularly with regards to improvement of pain.
- With the increasing demand on services and changing scope of practice of podiatrists, a way of monitoring cases collectively should be considered to allow improvements in care.

DISCLOSURE

C. Allen has nothing to disclose. A. Younger reports grants and personal fees from Wright Medical, grants and personal fees from Acumed PLC, grants from Synthes, personal fees from Axolotyl, grants and personal fees from Zimmer, and grants from Arthrex. A. Veljkovic is a paid speaker for Arthrex, Inc, and has participation in stocks or stock options of Therapia and Arthritis Innovation Corporation.

REFERENCES

1. Laughlin RT, Hartson JO, Wright DG. Training in foot and ankle surgery. Curr Opin Orthop 1996.
2. Hartnett DA, DeFroda SF, Ahmed SA, et al. Malpractice claims associated with foot surgery. Orthop Rev 2020;12:8439, 1, Providence : s.n.
3. Burton A, Aynardi MC, Aydogan U. Demographic distribution of foot and ankle surgeries among orthopaedic surgeons and podiatrists: a 10-year database retrospective study. Foot Ankle Spec 2020. https://doi.org/10.1177/1938640020910951.
4. Laxton C. Clinical audit of forefoot surgery performed by registered medical practitioners and podiatrists. J Public Health Med 1995;17:311–7, 3, Cambridge.
5. Finkel ML, McCarthy EG, Miller D. Podiatric Surgery: the need for a second opinion. Med Care 1982;20:862–70.
6. Chan JY, Truntzer JT, Gardner MJ, et al. Lower complication rate following ankle fracture fixation by orthopaedic surgeons versus podiatrists. J Am Acad Orthop Surg 2019;27:607–12.
7. Jakoi M, Old AB, O'Neill CA, et al. Influence of podiatry on orthopedic surgery at a level I trauma center. Orthopedics 2014;37:e571–5.
8. Chan JJ, Chan JC, Poeran J, et al. Surgeon type and outcomes after inpatient ankle arthrodesis and total ankle arthroplasty: a retrospective cohort study using the nationwide premier healthcare claims database. J Bone Joint Surg Am 2019;2:127–35.
9. Weiner JP, Steinwachs DM, Frank RG, et al. Elective foot surgery: relative roles of doctors of podiatric medicine and orthopedic surgeons. Am J Public Health 1987;77:987–92.
10. Harris RB, Harris JM, Hultman J, et al. Differences in costs of treatment for foot problems between podiatrists and orthopedic surgeons. Am J Manag Care 1997;3:1577–83.

Converting Ankle Arthrodesis to a Total Ankle Arthroplasty

J. Chris Coetzee, MD*, Fernando Raduan, MD,
Rebecca Stone McGaver, MS, ATC

KEYWORDS

- Ankle arthrodesis takedown • Ankle replacement • Painful fusion • Fusion conversion

---

KEY POINTS

- Ankle arthrodesis can give good clinical results, but there is strong evidence in the literature that over time the adjacent joints will develop degenerative changes, which could lead to significant secondary morbidity.
- Extending the fusion to a pantalar fusion has limited appeal because it severely limits function, and does not guarantee pain relief.
- Takedown of an ankle fusion and conversion to a total ankle replacement seems to be a reasonable approach in the correct environment.
- Absence of a distal fibula is a strong contraindication for a conversion to a TAA.

INTRODUCTION

The best definitive treatment of end-stage ankle arthritis has been debated in the literature for decades and even though ankle replacements are becoming more reliable and popular among the foot and ankle surgeons, a lot of experienced surgeons still treat their patients with fusions based on the overall good clinical results, high satisfaction rates, reliable pain relief, and good walking patterns.[1–3]

Despite that, ankle fusions are not without complications. Several patients complain about persistent pain around the ankle as a result of nonunion, malunion, or mal positioning of the joint. It is also known that younger patients submitted to ankle fusions more rapidly develop arthritis of the adjacent joints caused by added stress because the ankle is not moving.[2,4] These patients are unable to walk properly, have difficulties to perform their daily duties, and cannot participate in most active sports activities.[5]

The known long-term issues with ankle fusions could lead to further surgeries ranging from fusion revision, correcting alignment osteotomies, or also fusions of adjacent joints.[6] Arthrodesis to relieve the pain in the subtalar or talonavicular joints increases the morbidity and clinical limitations over time.[7]

Recent articles have shown that converting an ankle fusion to an ankle replacement has promising results and it could be the better option.[8–11]

HISTORY

Ankle arthritis is becoming more prevalent in the population as a result of the increasing number of injuries of the lower limbs. Tibia and ankle fractures, even when properly treated, may lead to ankle arthritis in the future.[12] Ankle instability is another frequent pathology that also leads to ankle arthritis.[13] Osteochondral defects on the talus or distal tibia can also result in ankle arthritis regardless of the treatment. In addition to these conditions, rheumatoid arthritis, hemophilia, hemochromatosis, and other clinical

---

Twin Cities Orthopedics, 2700 Vikings Circle, Eagan, MN 55121, USA
* Corresponding author.
E-mail address: jcc@tcomn.com

Orthop Clin N Am 52 (2021) 181–190
https://doi.org/10.1016/j.ocl.2020.12.005

conditions can also lead to degenerative changes in the ankle.[2,6,10,14]

Ankle (tibiotalar) range of motion (ROM) is somewhat limited compared with the knee, hip, or shoulder, and there is also movement generated from the adjacent foot joint. Because of that, fusing the tibiotalar joint has been the standard treatment for a long time. Because of the combination of satisfactory success rates and low morbidity with an ankle fusion, it continued to be the gold standard for a long time.[2,6,15] Total ankle replacements (TAR) became more popular over the past two decades. Initial barriers were that it was technically demanding, more expensive, and initially not as reliable as an ankle fusion.[1,16,17]

With time, improved hardware, and more refined techniques, the advantages of a joint replacements over a fusion are clearer. There is no consensus in the literature regarding what the gold standard treatment of end-stage ankle arthritis is, but replacements are certainly a good option.[18,19]

Multiple long-term follow-up studies of ankle fusions confirm several issues. Painful nonunions, malunions, and most important, progressive arthritis of adjacent joints are some of the problems that can affect those who had their ankles fused.[2,6,20,21]

In 2004, Greisberg and coworkers[8] published the first results in the literature and after converting 22 fused ankles to replacements, they were able to follow-up 19 ankles from 18 patients. Most of these patients had severe symptoms with significant restrictions of activities of daily living. The option of a Below Knee Amputation (BKA) versus a conversion to a total ankle arthroplasty (TAA) was part of the discussion.

Greisberg used a first-generation ankle replacement.[8] Ten ankles had intraoperative fractures on either or both malleoli and all but one healed without further procedures. The intraoperative ROM was 28° on average. After 39 months follow-up, five patients needed revisions for talar subsidence or for sustained pain. No mention is made about the technique for fusion other than to mention that five patients who had the lateral malleolus thinned or resection when the fusion was performed had a complicated course after arthroplasty. They presented with valgus tilting of the ankle and all needed additional interventions ranging from calcaneal osteotomy, medial column reconstruction, to below knee amputation. All three where the fibula was resected during the ankle fusion failed their ankle replacement and ended up with a BKA. The American Orthopedic Foot &

Ankle Society (AOFAS) score improved from 42 to 68; the final ROM was 26°; and 15 among the 18 patients were satisfied, stating they would go through the procedure again.

This was a landmark study but one of the main shortcomings of the procedure was that the first-generation Agility was the only implant on the market at the time. The talar component was a small triangular implant that covered about 25% to 30% of the talar bone surface. Especially in conversions of fusions the bone could be fairly soft, and subsidence was much more prevalent than in the modern revision components that covers most of the talar surface. Besides that, the syndesmosis needed to be fused, which is another important site for complications when the fusion was not achieved. These details must be considered when interpreting his results.

Five years later, Hintermann and coworkers[9] published results from 27 patients (29 ankles) submitted to a three-component ankle replacement. The patients AOFAS score improved from 34 to 70 on average. Patients with more than four previous procedures on the ankle or having had surgery less than 1 year before the conversion to ankle replacement had poorer results with more pain and worse functional values. The overall Visual Analog Scale (VAS) dropped from 7.5% to 1.8% and 89.6% of the patients had scores lower than 3. The final ROM was 25.5°, amounted to 56.7% of the unaffected contralateral side, and 82.7% of his patients were satisfied. They did not specify how the fusion was done, other than to say that the two patients that had the distal fibula excised during the fusion surgery failed their ankle replacement.

On 2015, Pellegrini and colleagues[11] published their results for 23 patients who had undergone conversion from nonunited, painful united, and malpositioned tibiotalar fusions to TAR. Two of those patients had their lateral malleolus resected at the time of the fusion, which required an allograft fibula when the conversion was performed to provide lateral stability for the replacement. Both these ankle replacements subsequently failed. They used three different replacement designs and were able to clinically and radiographically evaluate every patient after 33.1 months on average. Considering the information available on the patient's last follow-up appointment, 18 also had function score analysis. The Short Form-36 Health Survey increased from 37.7 to 56.4 in 18 patients, and the VAS dropped from 65.7 to 21.8 in 23 patients on average. The final ROM was 21.9°, measured clinically with goniometer. Among the 23 patients, 43% had low-grade complications (five superficial wound problems, two malleolar fractures, two tibial nerve, and one deep peroneal nerve irritation) and 4% had medium-grade complications (medial malleolar stress fracture) according to Glazebrook and colleagues[22] classification. Twenty patients (87%) had their original implants at the time of the final follow-up.

Huntington and coworkers[23] published results from five patients in 2016. They were conversions from nonunited tibiotalar fusions to a two-component fixed bearing replacement prosthesis. All patients had their fibula intact after the attempted fusion. After 21.3 months on average, his patients had a VAS of 3 and the AOFAS score was 82.6. ROM was 35° and four out of five patients were either satisfied or very satisfied with the procedure. The only dissatisfied patient stated that she was not happy with her rheumatoid arthritis course overall.

Preis and colleagues[10] presented results in 2017 and after an average of 54 months, they evaluated 18 patients submitted to fusion takedown and conversion to a three-component ankle replacement. They did not state how the fusion was done, or if the fibula was resected. None of their patients needed revision except for two cases of arthrofibrosis who needed open arthrolysis of their joints and the mobile polyethylene component was changed. Two patients had intraoperative medial malleolus fracture and three had delayed wound healing. The VAS dropped from 9 to 1.7 and the Short Form-36 physical and mental score increased from 34 and 49 to 74 and 75.5, respectively. AOFAS score improved from 23 to 68 postoperatively and the final ROM was 23.5° on average.

The encouraging results allow the option of offering patients an ankle replacement after years of painful fusions and functional limitations.

SURGICAL TECHNIQUE

Evaluating the preoperative radiographs is crucial for a successful surgery not only to determine the size of the implants but also to understand where the replacement should be inserted.

A fusion where the fibula was removed is a contraindication for replacement confirmed by all the previous studies. Arthroscopic fusions where no bone was removed, and the medial and lateral gutter was not fused, are the easiest to convert (**Fig. 1**). Conventional transfibular and/or flat cut fusions are much more difficult.

There are a few major principles to follow. The joint line should be established at, or as close as possible, to the original joint line. This is best done by using fluoroscopy in medial and lateral planes to determine the original joint level. There should be an aggressive medial and lateral gutter debridement. When the implants are in place, there should be excellent ROM. Motion will not improve as time goes by, so time zero should be more than what is needed. Consider removing complex hardware first, especially if there is a posterior tibial plate. The procedure is stressful enough, and the surgeon should have enough time to be comfortable with all scenarios.

Under general anesthesia and a peripheral nerve block, a sand bag is placed under the ipsilateral buttock so the foot is pointing to the zenith. A tourniquet is inflated to 280 mm Hg. A longitudinal 12-cm anterior incision is used. The anterior retinaculum is dissected along the lateral border of the anterior tibial tendon and the neurovascular bundle must be identified deeper to the extensor hallucis longus. The bundle is retracted laterally and the anterior tibial tendon is retracted medially.

The anterior aspect of the tibia and the talar neck are identified after subperiosteal dissection. A pin is inserted on the anterior tibial tuberosity and an extramedullary guide with a cutting block distally is used. The level of the joint is confirmed intraoperatively with fluoroscopy. Two pins are inserted through the cutting block on the anteromedial and anterolateral aspect of the distal tibia to control the swing of the saw blade medial and lateral. Anteroposterior fluoroscopy is used to confirm the distal tibial cut perpendicular to the long axis of the tibia. Lateral fluoroscopy is used to determine the level of the joint. In a perfect world one can still see the scar of the epiphysis, and the cut should be just distal to that.

The tibial cut is performed with an oscillating saw through the guide, perpendicular to the long axis of the tibial shaft. The vertical medial and lateral cuts are made with an end-cutting reciprocating saw, or a sagittal saw recreating the medial and lateral gutters. Fluoroscopy is essential for these steps. In a solidly fused ankle the traditional landmarks might not be there, and fluoroscopy helps to ensure the correct positioning of the gutter cuts, not to compromise the malleoli, but also not to cut into the talus.

The final cut, parallel to the tibia cut (if the ankle was fused in a good position), is performed 10 to 14 mm distal to the tibial cut on

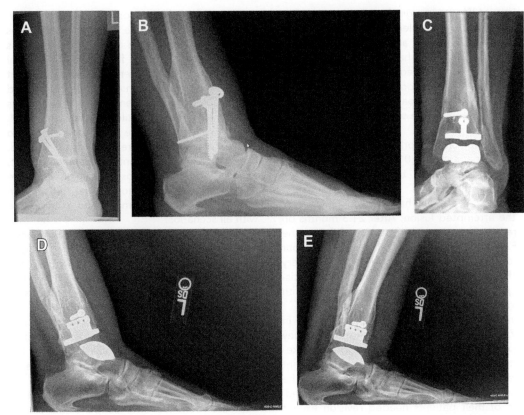

Fig. 1. (*A*, *B*) An arthroscopic ankle fusion done in 2001 for a 45-year-old patient with two medially placed screws. The medial and lateral gutter was not fused. Over time she developed increasing subtalar joint pain. (*C–E*) A conversion to an ankle replacement was done in 2014. These radiographs were done 6 years after the replacement. Anteroposterior (AP) view with no sign of subsidence of impingement (*C*). Excellent plantar and dorsiflexion (*D*, *E*).

the talus and the bone block from the fusion is removed. If any coronal plane deformity correction needs to be done, the correction is done at this stage, holding the foot on the desired position and doing the talar cut on the proper angulation. Two laminar spreaders are used at this stage. The bone block is removed and the rectangular space cleaned. The gutters must be free of any bone and soft tissues. Care must be taken when cleaning the posterior aspect of the joint, to avoid damage to the flexor hallucis longus and to the tibial nerve.

Trial spacers are inserted in the gap and the surgeon is able to check for ankle and hindfoot alignment and also for stability. If the ankle looks unstable after the insertion of spacers, ligament reconstruction should be performed after the definitive replacement is inserted. It is also possible at this stage to check for equines contracture and, if needed, a gastrocnemius or Achilles tendon lengthening.

The talus is prepared first with the appropriate guides, maintaining the foot in 90° and on neutral rotation. A flat cut is performed on the talus using the proper jig. With the conversions the talus is almost always a flat cut and no chamfer cuts are made. A poly spacer is inserted and the stability is checked once again, and in cases where there is only subtle instability one size bigger spacer is tried.

The width and depth of the tibial cut is measured and the proper tibial component is inserted from anterior to posterior keeping superior face of the tray in full contact with the tibial osteotomy. Previously the tibial component is mounted with the definitive poly because this is a constrained design ankle replacement. Radiographs must be performed at this stage to check the positioning of the components and to exclude intraoperative complications, such as lateral or media malleolar fractures.

At this point associated procedures, such as Achilles tendon lengthening, lateral or medial ligament repair or reconstruction, or malleolar or sliding calcaneal osteotomies, are performed. If the preoperative plan included subtalar or

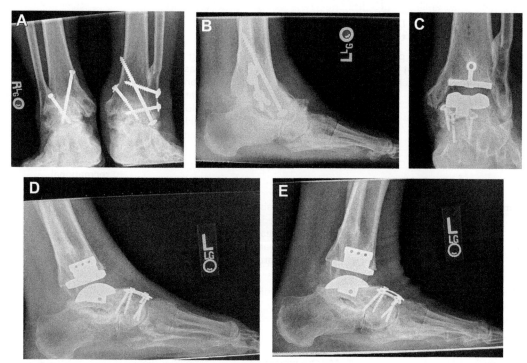

Fig. 2. (A) AP view of bilateral ankle fusions, both painful. Right caused by a nonunion, left caused by a malunion. (B) Lateral view shows a malunion of a left ankle fusion with the talus in plantar flexion. Eight years after the fusion there is severe talonavicular DJD. (C) AP view 4 years after a conversion to a TAA with excellent alignment of the ankle. (D, E) Plantar and dorsiflexion lateral radiographs showing satisfactory, not great, range of motion of the ankle. Also note the talonavicular fusion that was done at the time of the TAA because of advance DJD of the talo-navicular joint. One of the screws is broken, but it went on to an asymptomatic fusion.

talonavicular fusions, these should be done once the TAA is done to avoid malalignment. As a general rule the conversion to a replacement is done as a single procedure. However, if there is a significant malunion of the ankle fusion it could lead to severe talonavicular or subtalar arthritis that should be corrected at the same time. One of the most common malunions is a plantarflexed talus, which leads to severe talona-vicular degenerative joint disease (DJD). It that case a talonavicular fusion could be done once the ankle replacement is completed (Fig. 2).

POSTOPERATIVE MANAGEMENT

Patients were kept in a below-knee cast and were 50% weight bearing for 2 weeks. The cast and sutures were then removed, and a CAM boot used for the following 4 weeks. They continue to be 50% weight bearing and could move their ankle outside of the boot as often as comfortable. Physical therapy was started at 6 weeks and included ROM and strengthening exercises according to pain. Table 1 provides the full TAA rehabilitation protocol.

DISCUSSION

At this point, we have 51 patients and 52 ankles, with adequate medium-term follow-up to eval-uate outcomes clinically and radiologically. Fig. 3 gives an overview of the clinical outcomes as per the outcome scores used. There was essentially no difference in the Veterans Rand-12 Item Health Survey Mental and Physical scores between preoperative and postoperative. There was a statistically significant improvement in Ankle Osteoarthritis Scale Pain, Ankle Osteo-arthritis Scale Disability, and VAS Pain scores. The patient satisfaction rate was almost 90%.

These are encouraging results, but conversion from fusion to replacement is not without pitfalls and problems. Twelve of 52 (23%) had revision surgeries. This included two subsequent subtalar fusions for DJD, six cases that needed medial and/or lateral gutter debridement after a few years because of heterotopic bone formation, one cavus foot correction, one Achilles repair, one infected ankle that was removed and a cement spacer placed, and one unrelated toe amputation.

Table 1
Total ankle arthroplasty rehabilitation protocol

	Phase I: Day of Surgery to Week 6	Phase II: Week 6–8	Phase III: Week 8–16	Phase IV: Week 16–24
Objective	Healing, protection of joint replacement	Healing, protection of joint replacement	Swelling reduction, increase in ROM, neuromuscular re-education, develop baseline of ankle control/strength	Functional ROM, good strength, adequate proprioception for stable balance, normalize gait, tolerate full day of ADLs/work, return to reasonable recreational activities
Immobilization	Splint; after 2-wk follow-up visit: removable boot	Use of removable boot as needed Patient can wean to own footwear when they are comfortable		
Weight bearing status	PWB (50%), using knee scooter, crutches, and/or walker to aid with ambulation	Progress to weight bearing as tolerated	WBAT	Full, patient should exhibit normalized gait
Therapy		May be initiated toward the end of this phase, 1–2 times per week with a focus on swelling reduction, pain control, and early return of AROM, home care/exercise instructions for motion, pain/swelling control	1–2 times per week based on patient's initial presentation, frequency may be reduced as the patient exhibits good recovery and progress toward goals, instructions in home care and exercise to complement clinical care	1 time every 2–4 wk based on patient status and progression, to be discharged to an independent exercise program once goals are achieved, patient to be instructed in appropriate home exercise program
Rehabilitation program			Gradual progression is expected with ROM, strength, and function ROM: AROM, PROM, patient-directed stretching, joint mobilization (joint mobilization should focus on techniques for general talocrural distraction and facilitating dorsiflexion and plantarflexion) Techniques for inversion and eversion should be minimized and may	ROM: patient to achieve ≥10° of dorsiflexion and ≥40° of plantarflexion Patients with prior ankle fusion may be limited in ROM with 5° dorsiflexion and 30°–35° plantarflexion Strength: progression to body weight resistance exercises with goal of ability to perform a single leg heel raise Proprioception: patient should be

(continued on next page)

		Phase III: Week 8–16	Phase IV: Week 16–24
Phase I: Day of Surgery to Week 6	**Phase II: Week 6–8**		
		be contraindicated if the patient has had ancillary procedures, such as subtalar fusion or triple arthrodesis	instructed in proprioceptive drills that provide visual and surface challenges to balance
		The distal tibiofibular syndesmosis should not be mobilized	Agility: cone/stick drills, leg press plyometrics, soft landing drills
		Soft tissue techniques may be used for swelling reduction and scar tissue mobilization	Sports: before return to any running or jumping activity the patient must display a normalized gait and have strength to perform repetitive single leg heel raises
		Early goals for ROM are 5°–10° of dorsiflexion and 25°–30° of plantarflexion	
		Strength: techniques should begin with isometrics in 4 directions with progression to resistive band/isotonic strengthening for dorsiflexion and plantarflexion	
		Because of joint fusions, eversion and inversion strengthening should continue isometrically, bands should progress to heavy resistance as tolerated, swimming and biking allowed as tolerated	
		Proprioception: may begin with seated BAPS board and progress to standing balance assisted exercises as tolerated	
		Gait training: emphasis on smooth cadence, heel strike, and return to walking should be a primary focus	

Abbreviations: ADL, activities of daily living; AROM, active range of motion; BAPS, biomechanical ankle platform system; PROM, passive range of motion; PWB, partial weight bearing; WBAT, weight bearing as tolerated.

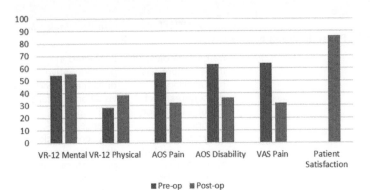

Fig. 3. Preoperative and postoperative outcomes scores. AOS, Ankle Osteoarthritis Scale; VR-12, Veterans Rand-12.

ROM varies from reasonable to excellent. The average dorsiflexion was 7° (0–15) and plantarflexion 20° (8–40).

The method of initial fusion and reason for fusion is important in decision making whether to do a conversion. Massive soft tissue injury at the original injury with significant soft tissue scarring limits the ability to regain motion with a conversion to replacement and should be a relative contraindication. The opposite side of the spectrum is an arthroscopic fusion for DJD secondary to primary arthritis with no soft tissue compromise. Especially if the medial and lateral gutters were not fused, one can expect an excellent result.

A more conventional transfibular fusion with flat cuts can limit the subsequent outcome.

Most of those fusions resulted in solid medial and lateral gutter fusions and some loss of height. If a replacement is done in this situation, care should be taken to do a wide and aggressive medial and lateral gutter debridement to allow free motion of the joint. Not opening the gutters enough could lead to early heterotopic bone formation and subsequent loss of motion (Fig. 4).

The original hardware choices can also affect the complexity of the conversion. The popular "home run screw" from posterior tibia to talus can pose significant challenges in removing. If there is significant hardware involved there is a case to be made to stage the replacement. First remove all the hardware, and at a later stage come back and do the TAA. A difficult hardware

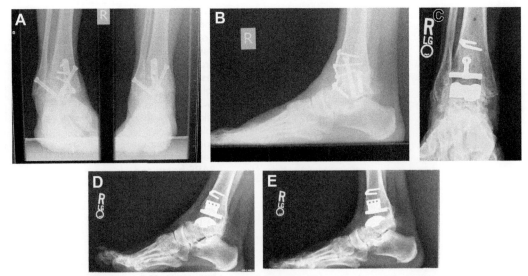

Fig. 4. (A, B) AP and lateral views of a complex ankle fusion that also fused the medial and lateral gutters. (C) AP view 5 years after fusions shows near ankylosis of the medial and lateral gutters caused by heterotopic bone formation. (D, E) Plantar and dorsiflexion laterals show most of the movement coming from the talonavicular and ST joints. This patient needed an aggressive medial and lateral gutter debridement to restore ROM. Preoperative and postoperative outcomes of fusions versus total ankle replacements. ST, Subtalar.

removal followed by a TAR can create a less than optimal surgical experience.

It is not uncommon to have an Achilles contracture after a fusion. There should be a low threshold to do an Achilles lengthening if needed.[24]

An ongoing concern is the apparent higher rate of implant subsidence in the patient group. In some of these cases the bone is soft on the tibial and talar side once the bone block is removed. Because of the fusion one does not have the usual dense subchondral bone of a normal ankle. Implant choice is important. The tibial and talar components should cover as much of the bone surface as possible and should have anterior and posterior cortical coverage.

SUMMARY

Conversion of a painful ankle fusion to a replacement is technically possible depending on how the fusion was done. The longer-term goal should be to develop criteria on when it is most appropriate and when one can expect the best outcomes.

From our study and prior studies in the literature there is some consensus that there are better outcomes with conversions for primary ankle DJD versus severe post-traumatic DJD. The method of fusion also plays a role in predicting TAA outcome. The less destructive fusions are easier to convert, with better long-term results.

From a technical perspective it is easier to use a flat cut instead of a chamfer cut talus for conversions. At this point there are no long-term published results and final verdict depends on looking at these patient groups over the next 10 to 15 years.

CLINICS CARE POINTS

- Most, if not all, ankle fusions lead to adjacent joint arthritis.
- Most of these become symptomatic.
- The options for treatment of adjacent joint arthritis after an ankle fusion are not well established.
- There is an increasing body of evidence that a conversion to an ankle replacement is a reasonable option for a painful ankle fusion.
- There should be a well-documented source of pain before a conversion is attempted. If there is no clear source of pain the likelihood of a good result with a fusion takedown is uncertain at best.

- A major soft tissue envelope compromise is a relative contraindication for a fusion takedown. It is unpredictable if reasonable ROM would be obtained.
- No fibula: no TAA.
- Insulin Depended Diabetes Mellitus (IDDM): no TAA.
- Beware of hardware; the more complicated the fusion hardware, the more complicated to remove. It might be best to stage the hardware removal and TAA.
- Try to avoid adjacent joint fusions at the time of the fusion takedown to replacement. Most of the adjacent joint pain might resolve or become manageable once the ankle joint moves and acts as a stress reliever for the other joints.
- Medial and lateral gutter debridement/exposure is critical. Without a wide-open gutter there is a high likelihood of excessive heterotopic bone that will limit motion and cause pain.
- Postoperative rehabilitation should be fairly aggressive to maintain intraoperative ROM.

DISCLOSURE

J.C. Coetzee: board or committee member for AAOS and American Orthopedic Foot and Ankle Society; paid consultant for Arthrex, Inc and Integra; paid presenter or speaker for Arthrex, Inc and Integra; IP royalties from Biomet, Arthrex, Inc, and Integra; publishing royalties, financial or material support from Elsevier; editorial or governing board at Foot and Ankle International; stock or stock options from Paragon, Crossroads, and Bio2 Technologies. F. Raduan: paid consultant for Arthrex. R.S. McGaver: nothing to disclose.

REFERENCES

1. Haddad SL, Coetzee JC, Estok R, et al. Intermediate and long-term outcomes of total ankle arthroplasty and ankle arthrodesis. A systematic review of the literature. J Bone Joint Surg Am 2007;89(9):1899–905.
2. Coester LM, Saltzman CL, Leupold J, et al. Long-term results following ankle arthrodesis for post-traumatic arthritis. J Bone Joint Surg Am 2001;83(2):219.
3. Atkinson HD, Daniels TR, Klejman S, et al. Pre- and postoperative gait analysis following conversion of tibiotalocalcaneal fusion to total ankle arthroplasty. Foot Ankle Int 2010;31(10):927–32.
4. Houdek MT, Wilke BK, Ryssman DB, et al. Radiographic and functional outcomes following bilateral ankle fusions. Foot Ankle Int 2014;35(12):1250–4.

5. Fuchs S, Sandmann C, Skwara A, et al. Quality of life 20 years after arthrodesis of the ankle. A study of adjacent joints. J Bone Joint Surg Br 2003; 85(7):994–8.

6. Lenz AL, Nichols JA, Roach KE, et al. Compensatory motion of the subtalar joint following tibiotalar arthrodesis: an in vivo dual-fluoroscopy imaging study. J Bone Joint Surg Am 2020;102(7):600–8.

7. Papa JA, Myerson MS. Pantalar and tibiotalocalcaneal arthrodesis for post-traumatic osteoarthrosis of the ankle and hindfoot. J Bone Joint Surg Am 1992;74(7):1042–9.

8. Greisberg J, Assal M, Flueckiger G, et al. Takedown of ankle fusion and conversion to total ankle replacement. Clin Orthop Relat Res 2004;424:80–8.

9. Hintermann B, Barg A, Knupp M, et al. Conversion of painful ankle arthrodesis to total ankle arthroplasty. J Bone Joint Surg Am 2009;91(4):850–8.

10. Preis M, Bailey T, Marchand LS, et al. Can a three-component prosthesis be used for conversion of painful ankle arthrodesis to total ankle replacement? Clin Orthop Relat Res 2017;475(9):2283–94.

11. Pellegrini MJ, Schiff AP, Adams SB Jr, et al. Conversion of tibiotalar arthrodesis to total ankle arthroplasty. J Bone Joint Surg Am 2015;97(24):2004–13.

12. Khlopas H, Khlopas A, Samuel LT, et al. Current concepts in osteoarthritis of the ankle: review. Surg Technol Int 2019;35:280–94.

13. Gribble PA, Bleakley CM, Caulfield BM, et al. 2016 consensus statement of the International Ankle Consortium: prevalence, impact and long-term consequences of lateral ankle sprains. Br J Sports Med 2016;50(24):1493–5.

14. Thomas RH, Daniels TR. Ankle arthritis. J Bone Joint Surg Am 2003;85(5):923–36.

15. Weatherall JM, Mroczek K, McLaurin T, et al. Post-traumatic ankle arthritis. Bull Hosp Jt Dis 2013;71(1):104–12.

16. Adukia V, Mangwani J, Issac R, et al. Current concepts in the management of ankle arthritis. J Clin Orthop Trauma 2020;11(3):388–98.

17. Bloch B, Srinivasan S, Mangwani J. Current concepts in the management of ankle osteoarthritis: a systematic review. J Foot Ankle Surg 2015;54(5):932–9.

18. Kim HJ, Suh DH, Yang JH, et al. Total ankle arthroplasty versus ankle arthrodesis for the treatment of end-stage ankle arthritis: a meta-analysis of comparative studies. Int Orthop 2017;41(1):101–9.

19. Veljkovic AN, Daniels TR, Glazebrook MA, et al. Outcomes of total ankle replacement, arthroscopic ankle arthrodesis, and open ankle arthrodesis for isolated non-deformed end-stage ankle arthritis. J Bone Joint Surg Am 2019;101(17):1523–9.

20. Henricson A, Jehpsson L, Carlsson Å, et al. Re-arthrodesis after primary ankle fusion: 134/1,716 cases from the Swedish Ankle Registry. Acta Orthop 2018;89(5):560–4.

21. Mills A, Fortin PT. Revision of the failed ankle fusion. Instr Course Lect 2019;68:275–86.

22. Glazebrook MA, Arsenault K, Dunbar M. Evidence-based classification of complications in total ankle arthroplasty. Foot Ankle Int 2009;30(10):945–9.

23. Huntington WP, Davis WH, Anderson R. Total ankle arthroplasty for the treatment of symptomatic nonunion following tibiotalar fusion. Foot Ankle Spec 2016;9(4):330–5.

24. Hintermann B, Barg A, Knupp M, et al. Conversion of painful ankle arthrodesis to total ankle arthroplasty. Surgical technique. J Bone Joint Surg Am 2010;92(Suppl 1 Pt 1):55–66.

Printed and bound by CPI Group (UK) Ltd, Croydon, CR0 4YY

08/05/2025

01864704-0013